VEGETARIAN AIR FRYER COOKBOOK 2021

60 Truly Healthy and Delicious Recipes with Low

Fat, Low Salt, and Zero Guilt, with Tips & Tricks to

Fry, Grill, Roast, and Bake

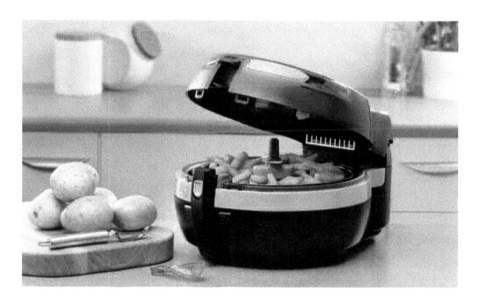

Thomas Patrick Blay

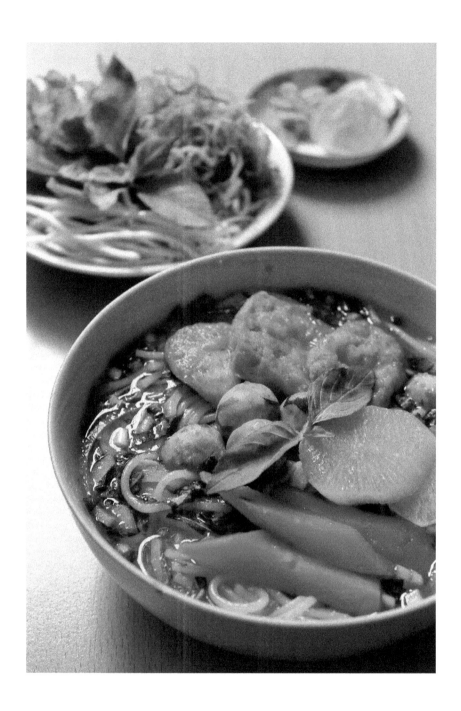

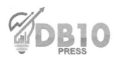

Table of Contents

WHAT CONTAINS AN AIR FRYER?

An air fryer isn't convoluted like other cooking apparatus. It contains a dish, a divider, preparing tin, twofold barbecue layer. The divider offers you the chance to cook two foods simultaneously.

Container fits well on the apparatus. There is a bushel which is put in the skillet. The bushel has a handle which permits you to shake your food during cooking without experiencing any difficulty.

There is a heating tin likewise which permits you to prepare merchandise and desserts like cookies and biscuits. The fixings which you need to cook put within the container, which consummately fits in the skillet.

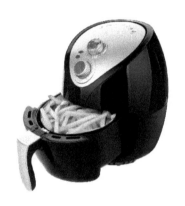

The fixings which you need to sear ought to be placed into the crate. At the point when you are going to evacuate the bushel, ensure that the dish is perched superficially on a level plane. Air fryer accompanies non-clingy surface and tempered steel.

WHAT IS THE MAIN PART OF AIR FRYER?

Manual Temperature

Only one out of every odd food needs equivalent temperature. This cooking cooker is allowing you the chance to work temperature of your own with the goal that food won't get over scorched. There is an auto arrangement nearly in each air fryer with the goal that you can without much of a stretch cook your ideal food.

Size of Tray

The size of the plate gives you the sum that the amount you are going to cook food. The Smaller plate is sufficient for one individual; on another hand greater plate is for more than one individual.

Size of Air Fryer

The diverse air fryer has a distinctive size of its own. Some are little, and some are large enough for an entire family. Some family has bigger space in their home, and some family doesn't.

So everybody can purchase this cooker for their decision. You can discover compact air fryer, which is especially helpful for the bustling individual who voyages a great deal.

Clean Easily

Cooking instruments are particularly hard to clean due to the oil of oil. Once in a while, it leaves a stain on the instrument, and it gets harmed.

In any case, the air fryer is liberated from it since it utilizes no oil to broil or cook any food. It tends to be put in the dishwasher effectively, and it is lightweight. In the event that you deal with the air fryer, you can utilize this fryer for quite a while.

Cost

The cost of this cooking cooker is very convenient. You can get it at a modest rate too. There is some air fryer which you can purchase at a modest rate and have a decent nature of this convenient cooking apparatus.

In any case, you ought to pick carefully in light of the fact that modest one isn't in every case great one and satisfy your requirements.

BENEFITS OF AIR FRYER

Consider the accompanying reasons why an air fryer may be directly for you:

Sound Cooking

Everybody cherishes the flavor of southern-style foods, yet numerous individuals must keep away from these for wellbeing reasons. In case you're hoping to bring down cholesterol or get more fit, your primary care physician may thank you for utilizing an air fryer. Air-fryers use up to 75 percent less oil than profound fryers, giving a solid option without giving up the season.

Speed of Cooking

The air fryer's little convection oven preheats and cooks more rapidly than an ordinary oven. You'll have scrumptious meals in a flurry, with less pause!

Green Cooking

Have you "made strides toward environmental friendliness?" Cooking with an air fryer can help. Most air fryers are energy proficient, and shorter cook times mean less generally power utilization.

Basic and Easy

Air fryers use basic controls, commonly two handles for cook time and temperature, or simple to peruse advanced showcase. You basically hurl the food in oil (whenever wanted), place it in the crate, and the air fryer wraps up.

Tidy Up Is a Breeze
The bushels and container of most air fryers are dishwashers alright for simple cleanup. Likewise, the encased idea of the air fryer

9

forestalls the splatters and spills related to profound searing and sautéing.

Safe

Coming up short on the huge oil tanks of conventional profound fryers, air fryers wipe out the danger of genuine consumes from spilled oil. Additionally, air fryers are structured with the goal that the outside doesn't turn out to be hazardously hot to the touch.

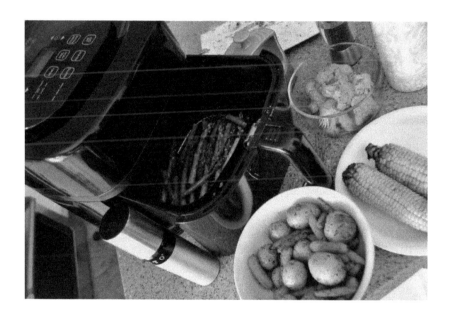

Other Health Benefits of Air Fryers

Air fryers are present-day cookers that utilization imaginative air dissemination and heat move innovation to sear and cook foods without oil or oil. On the off chance that this sounds unrealistic, at that point, you can settle your questions. Air fryers have reformed regular profound singing into a snappy, sound, and safe procedure. You would now be able to anticipate cooking most loved singed foods for your family without going with sentiments of blame. In the event that you've been considering putting resources into an air fryer, however, are not exactly sure, investigate the various advantages of utilizing air fryer in your kitchen.

Low Fat Healthy Cooking

One of the most significant advantages of air fryers is that we can appreciate delectable, dried up, fresh seared foods without going with oil, oil, and fat. The little oil makes a reviving appear differently in relation to the colossal puddles of oil that you'd have to use for profound fricasseeing foods. The manual will contain data about the various sorts of oils that can be utilized with the air fryer model being referred to. When all is said in done, air fryers use about 80% less oil (contrasted with traditional profound browning). For instance, 300 g of generally singed food will contain 37 g of fat while the equivalent 300 g of food will contain just 9 grams of fat when cooked in an air fryer.

It's totally brilliant to have the option to eat a more advantageous rendition of singed foods. Air singing lessens fat-loaded calories and subsequently diminishes inborn wellbeing dangers, including stoutness and so forth. Best of all, you're ready to eliminate the fat substance without settling on taste, surface, and flavor. Foods taste a lot of equivalent to they do on the off chance that they are expectedly pan-fried – you get the crunch, the searing, and the tempting smell too.

Quick Cooking: You can spare important time

The air fryer can be utilized for crunchy fries or firm chicken in practically no time. In contrast to convection ovens (numerous convection ovens take in any event 10 minutes to heat up to the craving temperature and afterward start the cooking procedure), the gadget needn't bother with time to heat up before beginning to broil food. Because of the high heat force, the viability of heat radiation is high, and foods begin cooking a lot quicker. The outside structures' prior and planning times are considerably quicker. French fries, for instance, can cook in as meager as 12 minutes and you can broil fish in a short time.

You can move solidified foods like chunks, potato wedges, and fries directly from the cooler into the fryer without sitting around idly on preheating. Nuts take around 10 minutes to become crunchy, toasty and fragrant. Furthermore, you can likewise reheat foods rapidly in air fryers – it takes around 10 minutes all things considered. This is a greatly improved choice of purchasing calorie-plagued prepared foods at the general store. Air fryers are especially helpful for cooking littler bits of food rapidly and no problem at all.

On the off chance that you have hungry children sitting tight for a meal, an air fryer can assist you with planning tasty foods truly quick! Additionally, the procedure is perfect and non-muddled on the grounds that all the browning occurs inside the fryer; no oil splatters to wipe up and clean. Regular stovetops accompany an uncovered surface and result in sleek fume beads that get kept on the ledge or in any event, roof. The cooker is ideal for individuals who need to cook in a hurry and eliminates time spent in the kitchen. All you have to clean is the trickle plate and cooking skillet, and you never again need to dispose of a huge amount of utilized oil. The flame broil, container, and bushel are completely worked to be dishwasher agreeable and made of non-stick material. It's a smart thought to drench them for quite a while before cleaning.

All things considered, the last we need is to remain around tidying up the kitchen when we have to race to work in a rush.

Basic and Easy to Use

Air fryers are anything but difficult to utilize and don't include any confounded dealing with. There are basically two kinds of air fryers accessible in the market: The bowl and mixing paddle model and the work base on the dribble plate model. Most air fryers utilize the work crate structure. The flexible temperature controls permit you to utilize various settings for various foods, and you can essentially adjust the cooking dish properly and overlap down the handle. You can utilize the blending oar to flip the food once in a short time to guarantee in any event, cooking. Truth be told, not normal for customary stove or gas cooking, you don't need to keep up a cautious watch over the container. At the point when you pull out the prospect (the food), the clock will naturally delay. At the point when you slide back the dish, the heating will continue from the latest relevant point of interest.

The main two fastens that you have to press the clock and the temperature, in any case, the procedure is, for the most part, programmed that requires negligible information. Indeed, a few models of air fryers even accompany customized settings for various foods. In the event that you're uncertain of the time or temperature, essentially press the right setting for the food that you're cooking. For your data, air fryers are worked to a meal, flame broil, and heat foods also. It offers adaptability and is easy to understand simultaneously. Actually, it resembles owning an oven, a barbecue, a skillet just as a toaster in a solitary gadget.

13

Numerous models of air fryers are planned with food separators so you can cook product meals on the double. You can spare a great deal of time without agonizing over the flavors getting stirred up. It's a smart thought to cook foods that require comparative temperature settings to cook simultaneously.

Safe to utilize

Not at all like traditional profound broiling that is laden with dangers of fire and spillage of hot oil, air fryers offer phenomenal security. The food cooks inside securely, and there is no risk of tipping over a dish of hot oil onto the floor. In addition, most models come outfitted with a programmed shutdown component that switches off the cooker when the food is cooked. This significantly lessens the danger of consuming or overheating food (Leaving hot oil on the stove or gas is hazardous as the oil may burst into flames). Air fryer cookers likewise have – non-slip feet' that forestall coincidental sliding and slipping. You can be certain that your fryer will never slide off the kitchen counter. Furthermore, the encased food chamber configuration guarantees that we appreciate a without splatter cooking encounter and don't need to fear getting burnt by hot oil. Reserve funds regarding time and cash

Since air fryers work quickly and utilize next to no oil, you can anticipate reserve funds regarding time just as cash. You save money on power use just as oil consumption. In addition, since the gadget closes itself down, there is no danger of energy wastage. Truth be told, you can even consider utilizing natural oils (they're typically progressively expensive contrasted with customary oils) since you need to utilize only a smidgen for cooking foods (pretty much a tablespoon full).

No Pollution

Numerous stoves, gas cookers, and so forth naturally include some type of ecological contamination. Air fryers come outfitted with cooling frameworks that keep the cooker liberated from pollution.

The heated air in the air-fryer is cooled and separated before being discharged into the air. The air channel likewise keeps the wet smell of oil from spreading around the kitchen. You can hope to appreciate crisp kitchen smells when cooking with an air fryer.

Scrumptious, Delicious and Even Cooking

The impartial heat move and configuration guarantee that food particles are heated uniformly. The food builds up a delicious smash superficially while the delicacy and succulence are held inside. Air fricasseeing jelly surface, flavor, and taste of foods. A touch of blending with the oar guarantees that no food is left uncooked. Oven and microwave cooked foods don't create a similar degree of crunch and freshness than an air fryer can deliver.

By and large, an air fryer is a protected, helpful, and flexible kitchen colleague which you can use to cook breakfast, lunch just as supper. Air fryers are an incredible venture for occupied guardians, wellbeing conscious individuals just as for the individuals who are consistently in a hurry.

You don't need to fear kids getting splattered with hot oil or the gadget slipping and sliding about on the kitchen counter. Above all, you presently have the alternative of getting a charge out of all-around cooked, succulent seared food without the orderly dangers of fat-loaded calories. In the present quick paced life and furious timetables, the air fryer is truly a much-needed refresher. They offer object free, quick, and solid cooking with insignificant exertion and supervision. You can cook your preferred foods without sweating over a hot, clingy stove. At whatever point you ache for singed food or feel too drained to even think about spending a large amount of time in the kitchen, you should simply turn on the air fryer cooker.

HOW TO USE AN AIR FRYER

There are four distinct stages during the utilization of any air fryer:

- ❖ Preparation Of The Food
- ❖ Preparation Of The Air Fryer
- ❖ Cooking In The Air Fryer
- ❖ Cleaning The Air Fryer

1) Preparation Of The Food

- ❖ Keeping the food from adhering to the fryer container, include absolute minimum oil.

- ❖ Let space between the food to permit the hot air to go through and cook from all sides. Utilize an aluminum foil paper as a separator.

- ❖ If you are utilizing marinated or slick fixings at that point, pat them dry. This will stay away from any splattering or overabundance smoke. Expel any oil/fat from the base of the fryer.

2) Preparation Of The Air Fryer

- ❖ Plug in the fryer and preheat it for around 5 minutes.

- ❖ Ensure that the air fryer cooker is sufficiently hot.

- ❖ Place the food things inside and abstain from congestion. Air must have the option to flow through all the sides of every food thing to cook it appropriately.

16

❖ If you are cooking pre-made foods, you can change the underlying oven temperature by 70 degrees and cut The cooking time down the middle.

3) Cooking In The Air Fryer

❖ While cooking little food, things like chicken wings or fries, attempt to shake the fryer around multiple times. Likewise, have a go at turning the food things at regular intervals to ensure an all-adjusted fry.

❖ If you are cooking high-fat food, you will find that it discharges fat in the base of the fryer. You would need to evacuate this fat in the wake of cooking.

4) Cleaning The Air Fryer

❖ After separating the food from the fryer, you should clean it appropriately to guarantee that the apparatus is in the top shape.

❖ You should clean the container and the skillet in the wake of using them. Many air fryers accompany dishwasher safe parts, which makes your work simple.

❖ However, if you have to physically clean the parts, at that point, absorb them hot water and include dishwashing cleanser. Following 10 minutes, clean them with a wipe while under the sink.

❖ This will guarantee that your fryer doesn't have any food particles obstructed in it, and your food's smell isn't caught in it.

❖ For cleaning the outside and within the fryer, utilize a delicate soggy fabric and dishwasher cleanser to spot clean the territory.

The air fryer will absolutely change your discernment about cooking. With its obvious quality and advantageous activity, it is unquestionably going to be one of your preferred kitchen cookers.

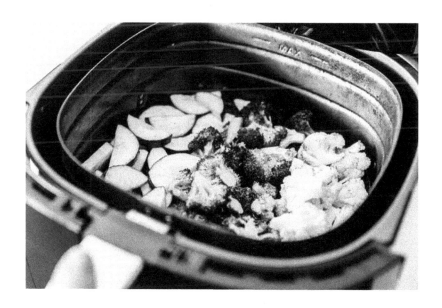

NORMAL MISTAKES WHICH ARE COMMITTED BY NEWBIES

Numerous purchasers lament in the wake of buying air fryer since they figure they would have purchased a superior air fryer at this cost. Once in a while, they don't purchase the air fryer, which satisfies their prerequisite.

Here are a few slip-ups which are submitted by new purchasers

Size:

The vast majority of the clients buy the wrong size air fryer. They purchase excessively huge or excessively little. You should remember that for whom and why you have to purchase an air fryer.

- ❖ If it is for the little family, at that point, purchase a little one.

- ❖ If you have a major family at that point, clearly purchase the huge one, so it spares your the cooking time.

- ❖ If you are a bustling individual and ventures a great deal, at that point, purchase the convenient one.

So be cautious about the size. You will lament on the off chance that you don't.

Numerous Features:

Few out of every odd air fryer has the same and all highlights. Some have numerous highlights, and some have essential highlights. In any case, you needn't bother with all the highlights regularly. Some new purchasers get intrigued by the new and alluring highlights, and they get it without pondering it. In the wake of getting it, they think twice about it.

So before purchasing any cooking cooker must reverify the rundown of highlights that you need and that you needn't bother with. Purchase that one which satisfies your prerequisites.

Overpaying:

If you are going to require an ideal and all around ok air fryer, at that point, you can burn through cash on that. Be that as it may, if you are going to utilize it for everyday schedule, at that point, don't go for costly one.

HOW TO CLEAN AN AIR FRYER

Making new and solid food from Air fryer is very simple and less tedious when contrasted and other profound fryers. In any case, air fryers likewise must be cleaned intermittently, for the most part, in the wake of utilizing it for some time.

Since air fryers don't require a great part of the oil while getting ready food, it is a characteristic procedure to clean an air fryer. By utilizing the best possible arrangement of materials and hardware, you can rapidly clean the air fryer. Underneath right now, make stride by-step strategies on the best way to clean an air fryer.

In the underneath article, we investigate materials required for cleaning the air fryer, at that point the means on the best way to clear all through the Air fryer, after which we investigate how to clean the Air Fryer bushel and dish materials.

At that point, we talk about reinstalling the parts back to where they ought to be, and afterward, we likewise talk about precautionary measures to be taken while cleaning Air fryer. At last, we will take some normally approached questions and offer responses for them and with some snappy video manages that let you know guidelines of cleaning Air fryer.

Prior to anything, you ought to comprehend that there are these five significant parts an Air fryer is comprised of. These materials are:

- ❖ Body or shell itself
- ❖ Air Fryer Pan
- ❖ Air Fryer bushel
- ❖ Air Fryer work

❖ Air Fryer exhaust vents

So once you know about the pieces of Air fryer, let us get jump into the cleaning procedure straightforwardly.

Materials Required for Cleaning Air Fryer

Before realizing how to clean an air fryer, let us investigate what are the materials required for cleaning an air fryer accurately.

Miniaturized scale Fiber fabric: Depending upon to what extent it has been that you have cleaned the air fryer cooker, the decision of material from assortments of Microfiber material can be chosen. There are numerous small scale fiber garments accessible in various bundles. It is encouraged to utilize microfiber fabric on the grounds that while cleaning the different pieces of Air fryer like work, container, and bin, there shouldn't be any smears or scratches framed on the outside of these materials. Between the medium to thin thickness will be sufficient to clear off the earth from the different components of Air fryer.

Non-rough scrubber wipes: The name may confound you a piece. However, yes, there are non-grating scrubber wipes accessible in the closest store, which has scrubber on one side and wipe on another side of them. The scrubber side is really to evacuate on the off chance that you have a greater amount of oil or oil adhered to the dish and isn't effortlessly expelled off. Wipe side is the thing that prescribed for cleaning the different pieces of the Air Fryer. These wipes joined with certain beads of fluid cleaner can try to please zones of Air fryer.

Cleaning Liquid: Again, the cleaning fluid is the one which really changes over that strong oil or food wastage was gentler and expels them from the Air dryer parts rapidly. This fluid, for the most part, consists of vinegar that assists with battling against those intense materials patched up broadcasting in real-time fryer parts.

Container brush: While choosing the skillet brush to clean the air fryer cooker, there are two things you should remember. One is that the fibers of the brush ought not to be that difficult that it might make scratches over the outside of the Air Fryer. Also is the length of the brush. It should go through each corner through the inward bit of the Air fryer rapidly. This will help you, whimsically, which will be depicted later in the article.

Paper clothes: These are again fundamental to spotless or dry the pieces of Air Fryer. Paper garments or tissue papers with no mellow abrasiveness can be utilized to clean the inward surfaces of Air fryer. You don't need to independently buy the paper towels in the event that you are as of now spending a great deal on purchasing wet non-rough garments.

Heating Powder: This is a discretionary decision. In the event that you think, there is a lot of smudgy parts inside the Air fryer and needs profound cleaning and drenching then you have to have preparing powder side by you to such an extent this can work productively and expel every one of those from those pieces of Air fryer totally.

Cleaning the In and Out of the Air-Fryer

So we should begin directly with the cleaning of the Air Fryer. To begin with, we will clear off within and outside of the Air Fryer first since they are very simpler to clean contrasted with the bushel and dish of the Air Fryer relying upon span, after which you are cleaning the Air Fryer. The following are the quite basic strides to clean inside and outside of the Air fryer.

❖ Unplug the Air fryer power supply.

❖ Remove the bin and dish portions of the Air Fryer tenderly with care.

❖ Once you expel the container and dish from the Air Fryer, you may see that there could be earth or buildup or oil of food aggregated. Nothing to stress, since this is very normal and can be handily expelled.

❖ Now flip around the Air fryer.

❖ With the assistance of cleaner you have bought or by making a Baking powder arrangement (3 gms. of preparing powder to 100ml of water), splash tenderly over the internal territories of the Air fryer.

❖ Let the arrangement enter through the buildup for 1 to 2 minutes

❖ Turn the Air Fryer topsy turvy once more, in this manner carrying it to the ordinary position.

❖ Wait for 30 minutes in the interim you can take a taste of espresso or complete some other pending works.

❖ After 30 minutes, rehash the means 4 to 8.

❖ Now put the container and bushel again into the Air Fryer at their separate positions.

❖ Fill the container with about 400ml of water so that in the following barely any means it can gather the buildups or soil from inside and furthermore give dampness.

❖ Connect the Air Fryer to the force source.

❖ Now work the Air Fryer at 200-degree celsius for around 20 minutes.

❖ After 20 minutes, you can expel the container and crate from the Air Fryer and mood killer the force supply, subsequently letting the Air Fryer chill off.

❖ Again flip around the Air Fryer when it is in tepid condition.

❖ You can expel the buildup of soil at the base of the Air Fryer with the assistance of wet garments or paper towels, as we recommended before. At that point, you can toss the water from the bushel or container gathered.

❖ Finally, when everything is done, you can unplug the Air Fryer from the force supply, and with the assistance of smaller scale fiber garments, you can clean the external surface.

❖ You can likewise utilize the cleaning arrangement or heating arrangement and shower it over the surface in the event that you feel it looks monstrous or has scratches. In any case, remember to clear off the earth again with a material.

Cleaning the Air Fryer Basket and Pan

Presently we come to generally significant or, on certain occasions, the most monotonous undertaking of all. The Air Fryer's most urgent parts are its crate and dish where you place all your tasty food things like Chicken or French fries or some other such stuff to cook. Since these parts are the person who is, for the most part, getting presented to the food things and the heat radiations from Air Fryer, it bodes well that these things will get filthy after some time and appropriate cleaning and upkeep of these materials now and again are very basic.

You can clean the Air Fryer crate and skillet first and afterward clean within and outside of the Air Fryer or the other way around whichever you are open to cleaning first.

- ❖ The initial step is to take out both container and work out from the Air fryer

- ❖ Then fill the Air fryer skillet with hot water once to which you can likewise include the cleaning arrangement, or the heating arrangement arranged dependent on its earth or oil to it.

- ❖ After filling the dish with water, let the bushel absorb the search for gold at least 10 minutes. This will help the materials connected to the container get disintegrated at the base of the dish.

- ❖ After a couple of moments, take the brush or non-rough wipe and clean all the sides of the container.

- ❖ Turn the bin topsy turvy and wipe the base piece of it tenderly with a non-rough brush or wipe

- After that, keep aside the crate and clean all the sides of a skillet with a non-grating brush.

- Finally, rub the surfaces of both containers and bin with paper towels or clammy material. You can likewise keep all the parts in a cold and dry spot for them to get dried totally.

Reinstalling all the Parts and Check the Air Fryer Functioning

Subsequent to cleaning all the pieces of Air fryer, next comes the reinstallation of parts and checking the air fryer working so as to be certain that it is working appropriately as it was previously.

When all the parts are dry, check for any of the rest of the buildups or the water forgot about on them and on the off chance that not, at that point, place all the parts in their separate positions. Additionally, ensure the electric string associating the air fryer to the force supply is perfect and isn't harmed.

At that point, place the Air Fryer to its unique position, which is upstanding on a level surface before you could begin cooking. There are vents accessible, which should remove the heat from the Air Fryer, subsequently keep up a protected good ways from the divider. Ensure the vents are looking towards an open region with the end goal that the heat can escape out rapidly.

At last, before beginning setting up your food in the air fryer in the wake of reinstalling all the parts, ensure that all the segments are in acceptable working condition and if at all they are harmed, contact the maker promptly and get them supplanted.

Signs for Next Maintenance

The following support or cleaning of the air fryer ought to be done promptly when you think it is looking foul, or it's been too long that you have utilized the air fryer. Beneath are some genuine considerations wherein you should hop in immediately to clean the pieces of Air Fryer.

1. At the point when you smell awful scent:

Air fryers are the freshest type of advancements in the field of cooking food. One may feel that profound fryers are better than air fryers as they are high on upkeep, however clearly, that isn't the situation. On the off chance that legitimate cleaning is done at a suitable time, air fryers could be your best accomplices while cooking food.

If you are utilizing an air fryer after quite a while and abruptly, you understand that an awful scent or foul smell is leaving the Air fryer when you take out the parts. At that point, that is your prompt first sign to clean the air fryer.

2. The white vapor leaving the air smoke:

Unquestionably, there are chances that you notice white smoke turning out from the vents of the air fryer when you turn it on. This could be a result of the accompanying reasons.

❖ You would have arranged greasy meals or greasy wiener meals and left the air fryer simply like that.

❖ You may have utilized over the top of oil for cooking a dish that isn't planned. Consequently, ensure you read the proprietor's manual and utilize the fitting measure of oil for planning singular dishes.

❖ Mostly, the low-fat materials are anything but difficult to cook through air fryer and inevitably are anything but difficult to get crispier. Thus while buying the crude materials or tidbits, ensure you look at the fat rate in them.

❖ If at all you can't avoid buying foods that are high in fat since you are kicking the bucket to set up that delectable dish, no stresses! Notwithstanding, ensure you clean the container and bin following use by the strategies referenced previously.

By following these straightforward advances, you can maintain a strategic distance from cost on upkeep and furthermore increment the solidness of air fryer.

3. Air pockets or Peeling Inside the Air Fryer:

There could be chances that before finding a good pace, grating materials shouldn't be utilized for cleaning reason; you may have used to the bin or dish portions of the air fryer. So since you have utilized them, you may see gurgling or stripping of the layer from the crate some portion of the air fryer.

Since there is the non-clingy covering over the container, thus there is nothing to stress over the food you admission. Nonetheless, the best suggestion is to contact the maker to the most punctual and get the issue settled.

4. Trouble in sliding the dish:

Once more, this may sound excess, yet there are chances that in the event that you haven't cleaned the air fryer in a drawn-out period of time and you are cooking through Air Fryer consecutive, at that point the aggregation of food or oil over within zone of the air fryer may happen.

The basic answer for this is to before you begin cooking for your next meal, clean the air fryer accurately as referenced above, and afterward feel free to cook your tasty dishes. Cleaning right now helps diminish your weight further.

Insurances to be Taken While Cleaning Air Fryer

Cleaning anything isn't a simple assignment, and when you are cleaning an air fryer on which you have contributed a considerable amount, you would prefer not to take any dangers or risks while cleaning it. Thus beneath are some basic precautionary measures taken while or in the wake of cleaning air fryer.

❖ When you are cleaning the pieces of Air fryer, make sure to deal with the parts with delicate consideration. Try not to hurry into things accordingly. Your closure of harm any of the parts.

❖ Use the preparing arrangement, when there is a great deal of soil living inside the air fryer or even on the crate and dish regions.

❖ Before and in the wake of cleaning the parts, ensure you check the ropes, all the pieces of the air fryer aren't harmed in any which ways.

❖ Never utilize the steel wire brush or scrubber to clean the pieces of the air fryer.

❖ Read the guidance manual or proprietor's manual appropriately before planning food.

❖ Don't utilize unnecessary oil for cooking food and attempt to cook the ideal amount of food without a moment's delay in an air fryer.

❖ Make sure that you clean the air fryer after each utilization with the goal that you don't need to burn through a lot of energy when it gets foul.

❖ Never submerge the parts which come in contact (Eg: Dashboard) to control supply in water. Utilize a soggy material to clean them appropriately.

THE DEEP FRYER AND THE AIR FRYER

A profound fryer is a cooking cooker that gives a generally sheltered approach to submerge food in the hot oil without the cook getting scorched. Cooking with a lot of oil can be perilous, as it will, in general, splatter and can cause genuine consumption. Oil is regularly heated to temperatures moving toward 280° to 400°F (140° to 200°C). As opposed to heat oil in a pot, it's a lot more secure to utilize a fryer to cook such foods.

This apparatus is comprised of an enormous tank, into which the oil is poured, and a container, which can be securely submerged into the oil after it has gotten hot enough. There are both business and home models. Business fryers are regular in drive-through eateries and are utilized to get ready French fries and different foods. A profound fryer isn't one of the most widely recognized home cooking apparatuses. However, it tends to be utilized to get ready singed foods at home.

When utilizing a profound fryer, the oil can normally be reused on various occasions, frequently upwards of 10 or 15. Either corn oil or vegetable oil are acceptable decisions; olive oil is commonly too costly to even consider using since a considerable amount of oil is required. Cooks can even keep the oil in the tank, as long as it will be kept in a cool spot and will be reused inside half a month.

There are numerous sorts of food that can be cooked in a fryer. Numerous individuals appreciate rotisserie French fries, sweet potato fries, mozzarella sticks, seared chicken, onion rings, potato tots, and numerous different kinds of food. A few gourmet experts guarantee that the ideal approach to cook a Thanksgiving turkey is to fry it profoundly. In profound fricasseeing, however, the food is submerged in oil, it doesn't commonly turn out to be excessively oily. Rather, the oil just infiltrates the food's surface, making it firm, while steaming within. Foods cooked along these lines frequently have numerous calories, be that as it may, in light of the fact that the outside or breading holds a great deal of the oil from cooking.

One of the most well-known dishes made in a profound fryer is the pan-fried Twinkie™, a development where a bite cake is dunked in hitter and southern style, with the goal that within liquefies and the outside is firm. This food may be scrumptious, yet very unfortunate. In any case, this treat would now be able to be found at numerous event congregations and different places all through the world, alongside pan-fried cookies and pieces of candy.

THE DIFFERENCES BETWEEN THE AIR FRYER AND THE DEEP FRYER

From the outset, profound fryers and air fryers appear to be very comparative. Both give customary food, (for example, veggies or bits of meat) a delectable taste and crunchy outside. Be that as it may, the technique a profound fryer utilizes (dunking food into a lot of hot oil) is vastly different from that of an air fryer, which covers the food with a tad of oil at that point shoots it with hot air.

On the off chance that you love conventional singed food, the profound fryer could be your most solid option. In case you're more wellbeing conscious and need to accomplish comparable outcomes without altogether surrendering that unmistakable seared taste and surface, an air fryer could be the ideal decision. You may even be pondering: Do air fryers fill in just as profound fryers? In case you're willing to surrender a slight measure of flavor and even surface to appreciate more advantageous singed foods, consider putting resources into an air fryer.

Regardless of whether you're looking for a profound fryer or an air fryer, you've most likely chosen a spending limit. You may likewise have considered certain highlights, for example, simple versatility or programmed temperature control. Looking at highlights, dependability after some time, general strength, and different components can assist you with narrowing down the accessible profound fryers and air fryers to locate what's directly for you.

1. Profound Fryers versus Air Fryers: Features

For certain consumers, a fryer's highlights (or absence of highlights) can be an integral factor. One element rich fryer we like is the Secura Triple Basket Electric Deep Fryer. This specific fryer incorporates a removable oil tank, an additional oil channel, flexible heat controls, a see-through window in the top, and a programmed clock.

As a rule, the two sorts of fryers share a few similitudes regarding highlights, especially with regards to advanced screens, flexible temperatures, and easy to use controls. Right now, banter about whether to get an air fryer versus profound fryer may boil down to only a couple of must-have highlights. The pricier the fryer, the more highlights it's probably going to have. For instance, you can locate a well-outfitted fryer with movable temperature control and a clock with a prepared sign and programmed shut-off. A few fryers even accompany cooking pre-sets to remove the mystery from The cooking time.

In the event that you acknowledge accommodation, you'll need to consider an air fryer with a straightforward touch activity and a helpful on/off switch. In case you're the sort to disregard food when it's cooking, a fryer with an advanced commencement clock and signal can be an incredible decision. Different highlights to consider incorporate simple to clean materials or fryers that accompany a formula book.

Southern-style food smells flavorful when it's cooking, yet it can likewise abandon a horrendous fragrance, particularly if it's been overcooked or consumed. In the event that you'd preferably stay away from this unsavory experience, search for a profound fryer with sufficient scent control (particularly ones with charcoal channels). Since cooking with all that oil can likewise be unwieldy — particularly when it's an ideal opportunity to tidy up — you may likewise consider a removable compartment with an oil pouring spout.

Other helpful highlights are cool-contact or collapsible handles and a computerized clock with an effectively discernible presentation screen. In the event that you need to remain in charge of your food all through the cooking procedure, search for a profound fryer with a customizable indoor regulator. A few units accompany show windows incorporated with their covers to let you take a look without opening up the top. Another component to consider is the unit's general force. A 1,600-watt power fryer probably won't appear that vastly different from a 1,800-watt dryer from the outset, yet the more impressive unit regularly heats and cooks food quicker.

2. Profound Fryers versus Air Fryers: The cooking time and Capacity

Perhaps the greatest contrast among air and profound fryers is their general size. Most air fryers are altogether littler than profound fryers, as their substance doesn't should be dunked into a lot of oil for profound searing. One model that has an incredible limit is the AIGEREK Digital Electric 3.2L air fryer. This ought to be adequate space for most home cooks.

In case you're searching for a fryer that is bound to fit on your counter, the air fryer is your most logical option. Try not to let the littler size moron you, however, as most air fryers have a lot of room for a better than average measure of food. You can, without much of a stretch, discover an air fryer with a 1.5 to 2-pound limit, which is all that anyone could need space to take care of two to four individuals. If you need the air fryer for an incidental bite or little meal, you can pull off a lower food limit, yet it's ideal for locating a bigger unit in case you're keen on making meals with the fryer.

Except if you plan on making the periodic broiled side dish, you'll need a profound fryer with enough ability to hold any food you want to cook. The Generally, the range is 2 to 12 cups, in spite of the fact that most of the profound fryers fall someplace in the center. While the serving size will shift dependent on singular needs, a 6 cup fryer is frequently enough for an OK measure of food for two individuals.

A few fryers accompany two huge bins or a blend of enormous and little bushels in the event that you want to make a little sum. Numerous profound fryers available today are enormous, requiring assigned counter space or capacity zone. Profound fryers are basic in café settings, but on the other hand, they're getting progressively famous among property holders.

The two sorts of fryers require some The cooking time to get your food pleasant and firm. In spite of the fact that they will, in general, be littler, air fryers commonly take longer in light of the fact that the food is cooked by hot air instead of oil. In a profound fryer, the hot oil heats up food quicker, bringing about speedier The cooking time.

3. Profound Fryers versus Air Fryers: Healthiness

Let's be honest — fryers aren't the most beneficial cooking cooker around. Another consideration as you're discussing an air fryer versus a profound fryer is calories. It's difficult to get those mouth-watering results (and the perfect measure of freshness) without utilizing oil, which implies more calories. Profound fryers work by utilizing a lot of oil, which the food is then dove into and expelled from. Then again, air fryers don't dunk food into hot tanks of oil. Despite the fact that you will place your food into a container with the air fryer, it's covered with a modest quantity of oil. The air fryer at that point blows hot air over it to cook the food.

If you're in the market for a dry fryer, which depends on heat as opposed to oil to cook food, you might need to consider one with Rapid Air Technology. This sort of innovation is fairly new available, and by and large, requires an insignificant measure of oil. A portion of the top air fryers available with this innovation utilizes something like 70 percent less oil than customary fryers.

In the event that you need a profound fryer rather, the Hamilton Beach 35034 Professional-Style Deep Fryer is pleasant in light of the fact that it has twofold crates with snares for simple depleting, so you get each and every drop of abundance oil off the outside of your food.

4. Profound Fryers versus Air Fryers: Maintenance and Reliability

If you don't care for high upkeep apparatuses, you'll be very content with a profound or air fryer. The two sorts of fryers normally keep going for quite a while absent a lot of exertion on your end. One choice that may speak to you is the GoWISE USA GW22621 Electric Air Fryer, which delivers an assortment of firm foods utilizing next to zero oil and won't use up every last cent.

The greatest protest among clients of the two sorts of fryers is that the plastic parts, for example, handles or even dishes to get overabundance oil, can sever or wear out after some time. In any case, these issues (on the off chance that they do happen by any stretch of the imagination) appear to collect following a couple of long periods of consistent use. The ideal approach to keep up the two sorts of fryers is to routinely investigate them, clean the units at customary interims, and intermittently check for indications of mileage. Most fryers (the two sorts) likewise require the oil to be depleted or sifted.

5. Profound Fryers versus Air Fryers: Price

You, by and large, get a great deal of value for your money with the two kinds of fryers. You'll pay more forthright for it is possible that one, yet the general dependability, low support after some time, and consistently flavorful outcomes make a fryer an incredible venture. It may appear as though profound fryers are more costly in light of the fact that they're a lot greater than air fryers. Be that as it may, most air fryers will, in general, cost more, particularly on the off chance that they're utilizing forefront innovation or inventive browning frameworks. A fair value run for a top-notch profound fryer is by and large somewhere in the range of $50 and $100. You can locate a balanced fryer for less, however, particularly on the off chance that it has a progressively minimized size.

Air fryers, then again, will, in general, range somewhere in the range of $100 and $200. In contrast to profound fryers, it's the particular innovation that the air fryer utilizes — as opposed to estimate — that directs the last cost. Most pricier models have Rapid Air innovation for quicker and increasingly proficient cooking (also less oil use when cooking). These units are additionally well-outfitted with highlights that numerous consumers find very valuable, from programmable settings to scent control and splendidly lit showcase screens with commencement clocks and alerts. If you're on a strict spending plan. However, this doesn't imply that you can't discover a consummately decent air fryer at a somewhat increasingly moderate cost. One ease alternative you may like is the VonShef Stainless Steel Deep Fryer, which just expenses $39.99.

THE SIMILARITIES BETWEEN THE AIR FRYER AND THE DEEP FRYER

Air Fryer versus Deep Fryer

Here we have set aside the effort to plunge into the subject of how air fryers and profound fryers analyze. What are their likenesses? What are the benefits of an air fryer? Does the profound fryer have a few favorable circumstances as well? We trust this article responds to every one of your inquiries on the clash of the air fryer versus profound fryer.

From the outset, air fryers and profound fryers could be viewed as being very comparable, and they are both after totally intended to cook food that is both scrumptious and has that seared food crunch. The strategy for how this outcome is accomplished is the place the air fryer and profound fryer contrast. The customary profound fryer includes sinking food into a pool of hot oil, oil that contains a great deal of fat. Air fryers attempt to decrease the oil required, some of the time to zero, to cook food, yet giving the ideal taste and surface. The air fryer expects to accomplish this by shooting the food with rapidly coursing hot air. Those with an eye on smart dieting will take note of the decrease in oil required is a significant advantage of the air fryer technique.

Both air fryers and profound fryers provide food for a scope of spending plans.

1. Air Fryer versus The Deep Fryer: Features

Here we'll lay out some key highlights you ought to consider during the way toward concluding which to purchase, an air fryer or profound fryer.

In the same way, like other kitchen apparatuses, both air fryers and profound fryers share some fundamental highlights, to be specific, digital screens, advanced or straightforward temperature controls, and an ergonomic structure. Air fryers go a lot in cost, and for the most part, the more costly, the more highlights it has. A few fryers even accompany cooking pre-sets for various food types.

Thinks to consider incorporate, does it have a clock with auto-shutdown? How simple are the materials to clean? Support of an air fryer is fairly basic, see our guide on the best way to think about the air fryer cooker here.

Profound fryers require various highlights, and as I would see it, the most significant interesting point when buying a profound fryer is smell control, search for one with a charcoal channel. Along these lines to the air fryer, you ought to consider that it is so natural to clean and keep up the profound fryer. Given the huge amounts of oil, cleaning, and care is additional tedious with a profound fryer.

Wellbeing is likewise of essential worry with a profound fryer, consider fryers that have cool-touch handles and a showcase window in the top.

2. Air Fryer versus Deep Fryer: Size and Cooking Capacity

We have recently expounded on the sizes and limits of air fryers accessible; see it here to enable you to choose what size you'll require.

This is one of the vast dividers in the skirmish of the air fryer versus profound fryer. Air fryers do regularly have a littler cooking limit, however, produces are tending to this issue with some presently propelling XXL ranges. Likewise, the way that the apparatus doesn't have to hold a huge sum of oil implies air fryers are commonly littler in size, occupying less counter room contrasted with a profound fryer.

We would prescribe going for the biggest air fryer your spending will permit as you'll presumably utilize it more than you anticipate. If you know you'll just utilize it for the odd little tidbit, there are a lot of littler ones available.

A 6 cup (size) profound fryer is commonly large enough for two individuals. Anyway, profound fryers do go in size from 2 to 12 cups. The bigger ones regularly accompanying 2 huge containers, instead of only one. Profound fryers are commonly less convenient than air fryers, so ensure you have enough counter space to forget about it fall time.

3. Air Fryer versus Deep Fryer: Health

Profound fryers aren't considered the most beneficial approach to cook your food, yet the vast majority of us are suckers for the food they produce. Air fryer makers guarantee that air cooking uses 80% less oil versus profound broiling. Clients of air fryers guarantee that the measure of oil required is even less; a few clients cook with no oil by any means. The huge decrease in oil utilized is the place the air fryer gets its a medical advantage over the profound fryer.

4. Air Fryer versus Deep Fryer: Maintenance and Reliability

Air fryers and profound fryers are both, for the most part, low kept up and solid. The fundamental consideration is how simple either is to clean, and this fluctuates by brand and model, get your work done on your picked model.

Both apparatus structures are all around tried now, and both ordinarily have a decent life expectancy, which is dependant on how frequently you use it, and how you care for it.

5. Air Fryer versus Deep Fryer: Price

Slicing directly to it, profound fryers simply win here, and they are commonly a little less expensive than a similar air fryer. Numerous conspicuous brands have a better than average air fryer for around $70, and given the medical advantages over a profound fryer, the little expense is justified, despite all the trouble.

6. Air Fryer versus Deep Fryer: Other considerations

Important is the air fryers flexibility, and it could be your lone home cooking cooker. You can see by the plans on our site that the air fryer can cook breakfast, lunch, and supper. Just as having the option to cook up a little treat now and once more.

AIR FRYER VEGETABLE RECIPES

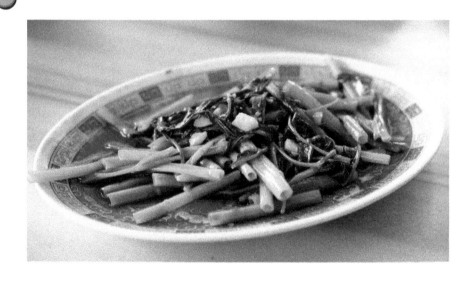

SPINACH PIE

Prep. time: 10 minutes The cooking time: 15 minutes The recipe servings: 4

Fixings	Guidelines
❖ ❖ 7 ounces flour ❖ 2 tablespoons spread 7ounces spinach ❖ tablespoon of olive oil 2 eggs ❖ tablespoons milk ❖ ounces curds ❖ Salt and dark pepper to the taste 1 yellow onion, hacked 	➤ In your food processor, blend flour in with spread, 1 egg, milk, salt and pepper, mix well, move to a bowl, massage, spread and leave for 10 minutes. ➤ Heat up a container with the oil over medium high heat, include onion and spinach, mix and cook for 2 minutes. ➤ Add salt, pepper, the rest of the egg and curds, mix well and take off heat. ➤ Divide mixture in 4 pieces, roll each piece, place on the base of a ramekin, include spinach filling over batter, place ramekins in the air fryer cooker's container and cook at 360 Deg. Fahrenheit for about 15 minutes. ➤ Serve warm,

46

	Enjoy the recipe!

✓ The nutritional facts: calories 250, fat 12, fiber 2, carbs 23, protein 12

BALSAMIC ARTICHOKES

Prep. time: 10 minutes The cooking time: 7 minutes The recipe servings: 4

Fixings	Guidelines
❖ 4 big artichokes, cut ❖ Salt and dark pepper to the taste ❖ 2 tablespoons lemon juice ❖ ¼ cup additional virgin olive oil ❖ 2 teaspoons of the balsamic vinegar ❖ 1 teaspoon of oregano, dried ❖ 2 garlic cloves, minced	➤ Season the artichokes with pepper, then rub them with half of the oil and half of the lemon juice, put them in the air fryer cooker and cook at 360 Deg. Fahrenheit for about 7 minutes. ➤ Meanwhile, in a bowl, blend the remainder of the lemon juice with vinegar, the rest of the oil, salt, pepper, garlic and oregano and mix quite well. ➤ Arrange artichokes on a platter, shower the balsamic vinaigrette over them and serve.

	Enjoy the recipe!

✓ The nutritional facts: calories 200, fat 3, fiber 6, carbs 12, protein 4

CHEESY ARTICHOKES

Prep. time: 10 minutes The cooking time: 6 minutes The recipe servings: 6

Fixings	Guidelines
❖ 14 ounces canned artichoke hearts ❖ 8 ounces cream cheddar ❖ 16 ounces parmesan cheddar, ground 10 ounces spinach ❖ ½ cup chicken stock ❖ 8 ounces mozzarella, destroyed ❖ ½ cup acrid cream ❖ 3 garlic cloves, minced ❖ ½ cup mayonnaise	➢ In a container that accommodates the air fryer cooker, blend artichokes in with stock, garlic, spinach, cream cheddar, sharp cream, onion powder and mayo, hurl, present in the air fryer cooker and cook at 350 Deg. Fahrenheit for about 6 minutes. ➢ Add mozzarella and parmesan, mix well and serve. Enjoy the recipe!

❖ teaspoon onion powder	

✓ The nutritional facts: calories 261, fat 12, fiber 2, carbs 12, protein 15

ARTICHOKES AND SPECIAL SAUCE

Prep. time: 10 minutes The cooking time: 6 minutes The recipe servings: 2

Fixings	Guidelines
❖ 2 artichokes, cut A sprinkle of olive oil ❖ 2 garlic cloves, minced ❖ 1 tablespoon lemon juice ❖ For the sauce: ❖ ¼ cup coconut oil ❖ ¼ cup additional virgin olive oil ❖ 3 anchovy fillets ❖ 3 garlic cloves	➤ In a bowl, blend artichokes in with oil, 2 garlic cloves and lemon juice, hurl well, move to the air fryer cooker, cook at 350 Deg. Fahrenheit for about 6 minutes and separation among plates. ➤ In your food processor, blend coconut oil with anchovy, 3 garlic cloves and olive oil, mix quite well, shower over artichokes and serve. Enjoy the recipe!

✓ The nutritional facts: calories 261, fat 4, fiber 7, carbs 20, protein 12

BEET SALAD AND PARSLEY DRESSING

Prep. time: 10 minutes: The cooking time: 14 minutes: The recipe servings: 4

Fixings	Guidelines
❖ 4beets	➤ Put beets in the air fryer cooker and cook them at 360 Deg. Fahrenheit for about 14 minutes.
❖ 2 tablespoons balsamic vinegar	
❖ A lot of parsley, hacked	➤ Meanwhile, in a bowl, blend parsley in with garlic, salt, pepper, olive oil and tricks and mix quite well.
❖ Salt and dark pepper to the taste	
❖ tablespoon additional virgin olive oil	➤ Transfer beets to a cutting load up, leave them to chill off, strip them, cut put them in a serving of mixed greens bowl.
❖ 1 garlic clove, hacked	
❖ tablespoons tricks	➤ Add vinegar, sprinkle the parsley dressing all finished and serve.

	Enjoy the recipe!

✓ The nutritional facts: calories 70, fat 2, fiber 1, carbs 6, protein 4

BEETS AND BLUE CHEESE SALAD

Prep. time: 10 minutes: The cooking time: 14 minutes: The recipe servings: 6

Fixings	Guidelines
❖ 6beets, stripped and quartered ❖ Salt and dark pepper to the taste	➢ Put beets in the air fryer cooker, cook them at 350 Deg. Fahrenheit for about 14 minutes and move them to a bowl.
❖ ¼ cup blue cheddar, disintegrated ❖ 1 tablespoon of olive oil	➢ Add blue cheddar, salt, pepper and oil, hurl and serve. Enjoy the recipe!

✓ The nutritional facts: calories 100, fat 4, fiber 4, carbs 10, protein 5

BEETS AND ARGULA SALAD

Prep. time: 10 minutes: The cooking time: 10 minutes: The recipe servings: 4

Fixings	Guidelines
❖ 1and ½ pounds beets, stripped and quarterd ❖ A sprinkle of olive oil ❖ teaspoons orange pizzazz, ground ❖ 2 tablespoons juice vinegar ❖ ½ cup squeezed orange ❖ tablespoons dark colored sugar ❖ 2 scallions, hacked ❖ teaspoons mustard ❖ 2 cups arugula	➢ Rub beets with the oil and squeezed orange, place them in the air fryer cooker and cook at 350 Deg. Fahrenheit for about 10 minutes. ➢ Transfer beet quarters to a bowl, include scallions, arugula and orange pizzazz and hurl. ➢ In a different bowl, blend sugar in with mustard and vinegar, whisk well, add to plate of mixed greens, hurl and serve. Enjoy the recipe!

✓ The nutritional facts: calories 121, fat 2, fiber 3, carbs 11, protein 4

BEET, TOMATO AND GOAT CHEESE MIX

Prep. time: 30 minutes: The cooking time: 14 minutes: The recipe servings: 8

Fixings	Guidelines
❖ 4 ounces goat cheddar, disintegrated ❖ 1 tablespoon balsamic vinegar Salt and dark pepper to the taste ❖ 2 tablespoons sugar ❖ pint blended cherry tomatoes, divided ❖ 2 ounces walnuts ❖ tablespoons olive oil 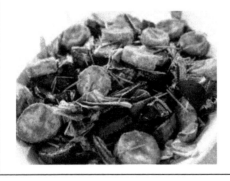	➤ Put beets in the air fryer cooker, season them with salt and pepper, cook at 350 Deg. Fahrenheit for about 14 minutes and move to a serving of mixed greens bowl. ➤ Add onion, cherry tomatoes and walnuts and hurl. ➤ In another bowl, blend vinegar in with sugar and oil, whisk well until sugar breaks up and add to serving of mixed greens. ➤ Also include goat cheddar, hurl and serve. Enjoy the recipe!

✓ The nutritional facts: calories 124, fat 7, fiber 5, carbs 12, protein 6

BROCCOLI SALAD

Prep. time: 10 minutes: The cooking time: 8 minutes: The recipe servings: 4

Fixings	Guidelines
❖ 1 broccoli head, florets isolated ❖ 1 tablespoon nut oil ❖ 6 garlic cloves, minced ❖ 1 tablespoon of the chinese rice wine vinegar ❖ Salt and dark pepper to the taste	➢ In a bowl, blend broccoli in with salt, pepper and half of the oil, hurl, move to the air fryer cooker and cook at 350 Deg. Fahrenheit for about 8 minutes, shaking the fryer midway. ➢ Transfer broccoli to a plate of mixed greens bowl, include the remainder of the nut oil, garlic and rice vinegar, hurl truly well and serve. Enjoy the recipe!

✓ The nutritional facts: calories 121, fat 3, fiber 4, carbs 4, protein 4

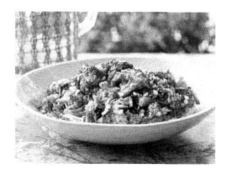

54

BRUSSELS SPROUTS AND TOMATOES MIX

Prep. time: 5 minutes: The cooking time: 10 minutes: The recipe servings: 4

Fixings	Guidelines
❖ Salt and dark pepper to the taste ❖ 6 cherry tomatoes, split ❖ ¼ cup green onions, cleaved ❖ 1 tablespoon of olive oil	➢ Season Brussels grows with salt and pepper, put them in the air fryer cooker and cook at 350 Deg. Fahrenheit for about 10 minutes. ➢ Transfer them to a bowl, include salt, pepper, cherry tomatoes, green onions and olive oil, hurl well and serve. Enjoy the recipe!

✓ The nutritional facts: calories 121, fat 4, fiber 4, carbs 11, protein 4

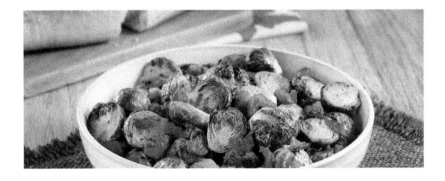

BRUSSELS SPROUTS AND BUTTER SAUCE

Prep. time: 4 minutes: The cooking time: 10 minutes: The recipe servings: 4

Fixings	Guidelines
❖ Salt and dark pepper to the taste ❖ ½ cup bacon, cooked and hacked ❖ 1 tablespoon mustard ❖ tablespoon spread ❖ tablespoons dill, finely hacked	➢ Put Brussels grows in the air fryer cooker and cook them at 350 Deg. Fahrenheit for about 10 minutes. ➢ Heat up a dish with the spread over medium high heat, include bacon, mustard and dill and whisk well. ➢ Divide Brussels grows on plates, shower spread sauce all finished and serve. Enjoy the recipe!

✓ The nutritional facts: calories 162, fat 8, fiber 8, carbs 14, protein 5

MUSHY BRUSSELS SPROUTS

Prep. time: 10 minutes The cooking time: 8 minutes The recipe servings: 4

Fixings	Guidelines
❖ 1 pound Brussels grows, washed Juice of 1 lemon ❖ Salt and dark pepper to the taste ❖ 2 tablespoons margarine ❖ 3 tablespoons parmesan, ground 	➤ Put Brussels grows in the air fryer cooker, cook them at 350 Deg. Fahrenheit for about 8 minutes and move them to a bowl. ➤ Heat up a container with the margarine over medium heat, include lemon squeeze, salt and pepper, whisk well and add to Brussels grows. ➤ Add parmesan, hurl until parmesan melts and serve. Enjoy the recipe!

✓ The nutritional facts: calories 152, fat 6, fiber 6, carbs 8, protein 12

FIERY CABBAGE

Prep. time: 10 minutes: The cooking time: 8 minutes: The recipe servings: 4

Fixings	Guidelines
❖ 1 cabbage, cut into 8 wedges ❖ 1 tablespoon sesame seed oil ❖ 1 carrots, ground ❖ ¼ cup apple juice vinegar ❖ ¼ cups squeezed apple ❖ ½ teaspoon cayenne pepper ❖ teaspoon red pepper drops, squashed	➢ In a skillet that accommodates the air fryer cooker, join cabbage with oil, carrot, vinegar, squeezed apple, cayenne and pepper chips, hurl, present in preheated air fryer and cook at 350 Deg. Fahrenheit for about 8 minutes. ➢ Divide cabbage blend on plates and serve. Enjoy the recipe!

✓ The nutritional facts: calories 100, fat 4, fiber 2, carbs 11, protein 7

SWEET BABY CARROTS DISH

Prep. time: 10 minutes: The cooking time: 10 minutes: The recipe servings: 4

Fixings	Guidelines
❖ 2cups infant carrots ❖ A spot of salt and dark pepper ❖ 1 tablespoon darker sugar ❖ ½ tablespoon margarine, softened	➢ In a dish that accommodates the air fryer cooker, blend infant carrots with margarine, salt, pepper and sugar, hurl, present in the air fryer cooker and cook at 350 Deg. Fahrenheit for about 10 minutes. ➢ Divide among plates and serve. Enjoy the recipe!

✓ The nutritional facts: calories 100, fat 2, fiber 3, carbs 7, protein 4

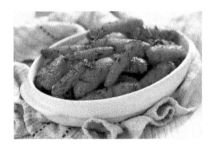

COLLARD GREENS MIX

Prep. time: 10 minutes: The cooking time: 10 minutes: The recipe servings: 4

Fixings	Guidelines
❖ 1bunch collard greens, cut	➤ In a dish that accommodates the air fryer cooker, blend oil, garlic, vinegar, onion and tomato puree and whisk.
❖ 2 tablespoons olive oil	
❖ tablespoons tomato puree	
❖ 1 yellow onion, hacked	➤ Add collard greens, salt, pepper and sugar, hurl, present in the air fryer cooker and cook at 320 Deg. Fahrenheit for about 10 minutes.
❖ garlic cloves, minced	
❖ Salt and dark pepper to the taste	
❖ 1 tablespoon balsamic vinegar	➤ Divide collard greens blend on plates and serve.
❖ 1 teaspoon sugar	Enjoy the recipe!

✓ The nutritional facts: calories 121, fat 3, fiber 3, carbs 7, protein 3

COLLARD GREENS AND TURKEY WINGS

Prep. time: 10 minutes: The cooking time: 20 minutes: The recipe servings: 6

Fixings	Guidelines
❖ sweet onion, hacked 2 smoked turkey wings	➢ Heat up a dish that accommodates the air fryer cooker with the oil over medium high heat, include onions, mix and cook for 2 minutes.
❖ 2 tablespoons olive oil 3 garlic cloves, minced	
❖ and ½ pounds collard greens, hacked	➢ Add garlic, greens, vinegar, salt, pepper, squashed red pepper, sugar and smoked turkey, present in preheated air fryer and cook at 350 Deg. Fahrenheit for about 15 minutes.
❖ Salt and dark pepper to the taste	
❖ tablespoons apple juice vinegar	
❖ 1 tablespoon dark colored sugar	➢ Divide greens and turkey on plates and serve.
❖ ½ teaspoon squashed red pepper	Enjoy the recipe!

✓ The nutritional facts: calories 262, fat 4, fiber 8, carbs 12, protein 4

HERBED EGGPLANT AND ZUCCHINI MIX

Prep. time: 10 minutes: The cooking time: 8 minutes: The recipe servings: 4

Fixings	Guidelines
❖ 1 eggplant, generally cubed ❖ 3 zucchinis, generally cubed ❖ 2 tablespoons lemon juice ❖ Salt and dark pepper to the taste ❖ 1 teaspoon thyme, dried ❖ teaspoon oregano, dried ❖ 3 tablespoons olive oil	➢ Put eggplant in a dish that accommodates the air fryer cooker, include zucchinis, lemon juice, salt, pepper, thyme, oregano and olive oil, hurl, present in the air fryer cooker and cook at 360 Deg. Fahrenheit for about 8 minutes. ➢ Divide among plates and serve immediately. Enjoy the recipe!

✓ The nutritional facts: calories 152, fat 5, fiber 7, carbs 19, protein 5

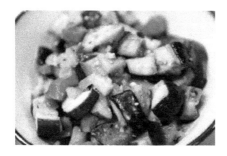

SEASONED FENNEL

Prep. time: 10 minutes: The cooking time: 8 minutes: The recipe servings: 4

Fixings	Guidelines
❖ 2 fennel bulbs, cut into quarters ❖ 3 tablespoons olive oil ❖ Salt and dark pepper to the taste ❖ 1 garlic clove, minced ❖ 1 red bean stew pepper, hacked ❖ ¾ cup veggie stock Juice from ½ lemon ❖ ¼ cup white wine ❖ ¼ cup parmesan, ground	➤ Heat up a container that accommodates the air fryer cooker with the oil over medium high heat, include garlic and stew pepper, mix and cook for 2 minutes. ➤ Add fennel, salt, pepper, stock, wine, lemon juice, and parmesan, hurl to cover, present in the air fryer cooker and cook at 350 Deg. Fahrenheit for about 6 minutes. ➤ Divide among plates and serve immediately. Enjoy the recipe!

✓ The nutritional facts: calories 100, fat 4, fiber 8, carbs 4, protein 4

OKRA AND CORN SALAD

Prep. time: 10 minutes: The cooking time: 12 minutes: The recipe servings: 6

Fixings	Guidelines
❖ 1 pound okra, cut 6 scallions, slashed	➤ Heat up a skillet that accommodates the air fryer cooker with the oil over medium high heat, include scallions and ringer peppers, mix and cook for 5 minutes.
❖ 3 green ringer peppers, slashed	
❖ Salt and dark pepper to the taste	➤ Add okra, salt, pepper, sugar, tomatoes and corn, mix, present in the air fryer cooker and cook at 360 Deg. Fahrenheit for about 7 minutes.
❖ 2 tablespoons olive oil	
❖ 1 teaspoon sugar	
❖ 28 ounces canned tomatoes, slashed	➤ Divide okra blend on plates and serve warm.
❖ 1 cup con	Enjoy the recipe!

✓ The nutritional facts: calories 152, fat 4, fiber 3, carbs 18, protein 4

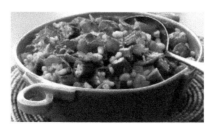

AIR FRIED LEEKS

Prep. time: 10 minutes: The cooking time: 7 minutes: The recipe servings: 4

Fixings	Guidelines
❖ 4 leeks, washed, closes cut off and divided ❖ Salt and dark pepper to the taste ❖ 1 tablespoon margarine, softened ❖ 1 tablespoon lemon juice	➢ Rub leeks with dissolved spread, season with salt and pepper, put in the air fryer cooker and cook at 350 Deg. Fahrenheit for about 7 minutes. ➢ Arrange on a platter, shower lemon squeeze all finished and serve. Enjoy the recipe!

✓ The nutritional facts: calories 100, fat 4, fiber 2, carbs 6, protein 2

FIRM POTATOES AND PARSLEY

Prep. time: 10 minutes: The cooking time: 10 minutes: The recipe servings: 4

Fixings	Guidelines
❖ pound gold potatoes, cut into wedges ❖ Salt and dark pepper to the taste ❖ tablespoons olive Juice from ½ lemon ❖ ¼ cup parsley leaves, hacked	➤ Rub potatoes with salt, pepper, lemon juice and olive oil, put them in the air fryer cooker and cook at 350 Deg. Fahrenheit for about 10 minutes. ➤ Divide among plates, sprinkle parsley on top and serve. Enjoy the recipe!

✓ The nutritional facts: calories 152, fat 3, fiber 7, carbs 17, protein 4

INDIAN TURNIPS SALAD

Prep. time: 10 minutes: The cooking time: 12 minutes: The recipe servings: 4

Fixings	Guidelines
❖ 20 ounces turnips, stripped and slashed ❖ 1 teaspoon garlic, minced ❖ 1 teaspoon ginger, ground ❖ 2 yellow onions, slashed ❖ 2 tomatoes, cleaved ❖ 1 teaspoon cumin, ground ❖ 1 teaspoon coriander, ground ❖ 2 green chilies, slashed ❖ ½ teaspoon turmeric powder ❖ 2 tablespoons margarine ❖ Salt and dark pepper to the taste ❖ A bunch coriander leaves,	➢ Heat up a skillet that accommodates the air fryer cooker with the margarine, liquefy it, include green chilies, garlic and ginger, mix and cook for 1 moment. ➢ Add onions, salt, pepper, tomatoes, turmeric, cumin, ground coriander and turnips, mix, present in the air fryer cooker and cook at 350 Deg. Fahrenheit for about 10 minutes. ➢ Divide among plates, sprinkle new coriander on top and serve. Enjoy the recipe!

slashed	

✓ The nutritional facts: calories 100, fat 3, fiber 6, carbs 12, protein 4

STRAIGHTFORWARD STUFFED TOMATOES

Prep. time: 10 minutes: The cooking time: 15 minutes: The recipe servings: 4

Fixings	Guidelines
❖ 4 tomatoes, finishes cut off and mash scooped and hacked ❖ Salt and dark pepper to the taste ❖ yellow onion, cleaved ❖ 1 tablespoon spread ❖ Tablespoons celery, cleaved ❖ ½ cup mushrooms, cleaved ❖ 1 tablespoon bread pieces ❖ 1 cup curds ❖ ¼ teaspoon caraway seeds	➢ Heat up a container with the spread over medium heat, liquefy it, include onion and celery, mix and cook for 3 minutes. ➢ Add tomato mash and mushrooms, mix and cook for brief more. ➢ Add salt, pepper, disintegrated bread, cheddar, caraway seeds and parsley, mix, cook for 4 minutes more and take off heat. ➢ Stuff tomatoes with this blend, place them in the air fryer cooker and cook at 350 Deg. Fahrenheit for about 8 minutes.

❖ 1 tablespoon parsley, cleaved	➤ Divide stuffed tomatoes on plates and serve. Enjoy the recipe!

✓ The nutritional facts: calories 143, fat 4, fiber 6, carbs 4, protein 4

INDIAN POTATOES

Prep. time: 10 minutes: The cooking time: 12 minutes: The recipe servings: 4

Fixings	Guidelines
❖ 1 tablespoon of the coriander seeds ❖ 1 tablespoon of the cumin seeds ❖ Salt and dark pepper to the taste ❖ ½ teaspoon turmeric powder ❖ ½ teaspoon red bean stew powder	➤ Heat up a container that accommodates the air fryer cooker with the oil over medium heat, include coriander and cumin seeds, mix and cook for 2 minutes. ➤ Add salt, pepper, turmeric, bean stew powder, pomegranate powder, mango, fenugreek and potatoes, hurl, present in the air fryer cooker and cook at 360 Deg. Fahrenheit for about 10 minutes.

❖ 1 teaspoon pomegranate powder	➤ Divide among plates and serve hot.
❖ 1 tablespoon cured mango, hacked	Enjoy the recipe!
❖ 2 teaspoons fenugreek, dried	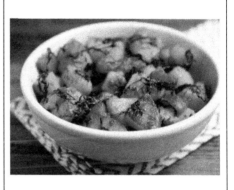
❖ 5 potatoes, bubbled, stripped and cubed	
❖ 2 tablespoons olive oil	

✓ The nutritional facts: calories 251, fat 7, fiber 4, carbs 12, protein 7

BROCCOLI AND TOMATOES AIR FRIED STEW

Prep. time: 10 minutes: The cooking time: 20 minutes: The recipe servings: 4

Fixings	Guidelines
❖ 1 broccoli head, florets isolated ❖ 2 teaspoons coriander seeds ❖ 1 tablespoon of olive oil ❖ 1 yellow onion, hacked	➤ Heat up a dish that accommodates the air fryer cooker with the oil over medium heat, include onions, salt, pepper and red pepper, mix and cook for 7 minutes. ➤ Add ginger, garlic, coriander seeds, tomatoes and broccoli,

Fixings	Guidelines
❖ Salt and dark pepper to the taste	mix, present in the air fryer cooker and cook at 360 Deg. Fahrenheit for about 12 minutes.
❖ A touch of red pepper, squashed	➢ Divide into bowls and serve.
❖ 1 little ginger piece, hacked	Enjoy the recipe!
❖ 1 garlic clove, minced	
❖ 28 ounces canned tomatoes, pureed	

✓ The nutritional facts: calories 150, fat 4, fiber 2, carbs 7, protein 12

COLLARD GREENS AND BACON

Prep. time: 10 minutes: The cooking time: 12 minutes: The recipe servings: 4

Fixings	Guidelines
❖ 1pound collard greens	➢ Heat up a dish that accommodates the air fryer cooker over medium heat, include bacon, mix and cook 1-2 minutes
❖ 3 bacon strips, hacked	
❖ ¼ cup cherry tomatoes, split	➢ Add tomatoes, collard

❖ 1 tablespoon apple juice vinegar ❖ 2 tablespoons chicken stock ❖ Salt and dark pepper to the taste	greens, vinegar, stock, salt and pepper, mix, present in the air fryer cooker and cook at 320 Deg. Fahrenheit for about 10 minutes. ➤ Divide among plates and serve. Enjoy the recipe!

✓ The nutritional facts: calories 120, fat 3, fiber 1, carbs 3, protein 7

SESAME MUSTARD GREENS

Prep. time: 10 minutes: The cooking time: 11 minutes: The recipe servings: 4

Fixings	Guidelines
❖ 2garlic cloves, minced ❖ 1 pound mustard greens, torn ❖ 1 tablespoon of olive oil ❖ ½ cup yellow onion, cut ❖ Salt and dark pepper to the taste	➤ Heat up a dish that accommodates the air fryer cooker with the oil over medium heat, include onions, mix and dark colored them for 5 minutes. ➤ Add garlic, stock, greens, salt and pepper, mix, present in the air fryer cooker and cook at 350 Deg. Fahrenheit for about 6 minutes.

❖ 3 tablespoons veggie stock ❖ ¼ teaspoon dull sesame oil	➢ Add sesame oil, hurl to cover, separate among plates and serve. Enjoy the recipe!

✓ The nutritional facts: calories 120, fat 3, fiber 1, carbs 3, protein 7

RADISH HASH

Prep. time: 10 minutes: The cooking time: 7 minutes: The recipe servings: 4

Fixings	Guidelines
❖ ½ teaspoon onion powder ❖ 1 pound radishes, cut ❖ ½ teaspoon garlic powder ❖ Salt and dark pepper to the taste ❖ 4 eggs ❖ 1/3 cup parmesan, ground	➢ In a bowl, blend radishes in with salt, pepper, onion and garlic powder, eggs and parmesan and mix well. ➢ Transfer radishes to a container that accommodates the air fryer cooker and cook at 350 Deg. Fahrenheit for about 7 minutes. ➢ Divide hash on plates and serve. Enjoy the recipe!

✓ The nutritional facts: calories 80, fat 5, fiber 2, carbs 5, protein 7

DELIGHTFUL ZUCCHINI MIX

Prep. time: 10 minutes: The cooking time: 14 minutes: The recipe servings: 6

Fixings	Guidelines
❖ 6 zucchinis, split and afterward cut ❖ Salt and dark pepper to the taste ❖ 1 tablespoon margarine ❖ teaspoon oregano, dried ❖ ½ cup yellow onion, cleaved ❖ 3 garlic cloves, minced ❖ ounces parmesan, ground ❖ ¾cup overwhelming cream	➢ Heat up a container that accommodates the air fryer cooker with the spread over medium high heat, include onion, mix and cook for 4 minutes. ➢ Add garlic, zucchinis, oregano, salt, pepper and overwhelming cream, hurl, present in the air fryer cooker and cook at 350 Deg. Fahrenheit for about 10 minutes. ➢ Add parmesan, mix, partition among plates and serve. Enjoy the recipe!

SWISS CHARD AND SAUSAGE

Prep. time: 10 minutes: The cooking time: 20 minutes: The recipe servings: 8

Fixings	Guidelines
❖ 8 cups Swiss chard, cleaved ❖ ½ cup onion, cleaved ❖ 1 tablespoon of olive oil ❖ 1 garlic clove, minced ❖ Salt and dark pepper to the taste ❖ 3 eggs ❖ 2 cups ricotta cheddar ❖ 1 cup mozzarella, destroyed ❖ A spot of nutmeg ❖ ¼ cup parmesan, ground	➤ Heat up a skillet that accommodates the air fryer cooker with the oil over medium heat, include onions, garlic, Swiss chard, salt, pepper and nutmeg, mix, cook for 2 minutes and take off heat. ➤ In a bowl, whisk eggs with mozzarella, parmesan and ricotta, mix, pour over Swiss chard blend, hurl, present in the air fryer cooker and cook at 320 Deg. Fahrenheit for about 17 minutes. ➤ Divide among plates and serve. Enjoy the recipe!

❖ 1 pound wiener, hacked	

✓ The nutritional facts: calories 332, fat 13, fiber 3, carbs 14, protein 23

SWISS CHARD SALAD

Prep. time: 10 minutes: The cooking time: 13 minutes: The recipe servings: 4

Fixings	Guidelines
❖ 1 bundle Swiss chard, torn ❖ 2 tablespoons olive oil ❖ 1 little yellow onion, slashed ❖ A spot of red pepper chips ❖ ¼ cup pine nuts, toasted ❖ ¼ cup raisins ❖ 1 tablespoon balsamic vinegar ❖ Salt and dark pepper to the taste	➢ Heat up a skillet that accommodates the air fryer cooker with the oil over medium heat, include chard and onions, mix and cook for 5 minutes. ➢ Add salt, pepper, pepper drops, raisins, pine nuts and vinegar, mix, present in the air fryer cooker and cook at 350 Deg. Fahrenheit for about 8 minutes. ➢ Divide among plates and serve. Enjoy the recipe!

✓ The nutritional facts: calories 120, fat 2, fiber 1, carbs 8, protein 8

SPANISH GREENS

Prep. time: 10 minutes: The cooking time: 8 minutes: The recipe servings: 4

Fixings	Guidelines
❖ 1 apple, cored and slashed ❖ 1 yellow onion, cut ❖ 3 tablespoons olive oil ❖ ¼ cup raisins ❖ 6 garlic cloves, slashed ❖ ¼ cup pine nuts, toasted ❖ ¼ cup balsamic vinegar ❖ 5 cups blended spinach and chard ❖ Salt and dark pepper to the taste ❖ A spot of nutmeg	➤ Heat up a skillet that accommodates the air fryer cooker with the oil over medium high heat, include onion, mix and cook for 3 minutes. ➤ Add apple, garlic, raisins, vinegar, blended spinach and chard, nutmeg, salt and pepper, mix, present in preheated air fryer and cook at 350 Deg. Fahrenheit for about 5 minutes. ➤ Divide between the plates, and sprinkle pine nuts on top and serve. Enjoy the recipe!

✓ The nutritional facts: calories 120, fat 1, fiber 2, carbs 3, protein 6

ENHANCED AIR FRIED TOMATOES

Prep. time: 10 minutes: The cooking time: 15: The recipe servings: 8

Fixings	Guidelines
❖ jalapeno pepper, slashed ❖ 4 garlic cloves, minced ❖ pounds cherry tomatoes, divided ❖ Salt and dark pepper to the taste ❖ ¼ cup olive oil ❖ ½ teaspoon oregano, dried ❖ ¼ cup basil, slashed ❖ ½ cup parmesan, ground	➢ In a bowl, blend tomatoes in with garlic, jalapeno, season with salt, pepper and oregano and sprinkle the oil, hurl to cover, present in the air fryer cooker and cook at 380 Deg. Fahrenheit for about 15 minutes. ➢ Transfer tomatoes to a bowl, include basil and parmesan, hurl and serve. Enjoy the recipe!

✓ The nutritional facts: calories 140, fat 2, fiber 2, carbs 6, protein 8

ITALIAN EGGPLANT STEW

Prep. time: 10 minutes: The cooking time: 15 minutes: The recipe servings: 4

Fixings	Guidelines
❖ red onion, hacked ❖ garlic cloves, hacked ❖ 1 bundle parsley, slashed ❖ Salt and dark pepper to the taste ❖ 1 teaspoon oregano, dried ❖ eggplants, cut into medium pieces ❖ 2 tablespoons olive oil ❖ 2 tablespoons tricks, slashed ❖ 1 bunch green olives, hollowed and cut ❖ 5 tomatoes, hacked ❖ tablespoons herb vinegar	➢ Heat up a dish that accommodates the air fryer cooker with the oil over medium heat, include eggplant, oregano, salt and pepper, mix and cook for 5 minutes. ➢ Add garlic, onion, parsley, tricks, olives, vinegar and tomatoes, mix, present in the air fryer cooker and cook at 360 Deg. Fahrenheit for about 15 minutes. ➢ Divide into bowls and serve. Enjoy the recipe! 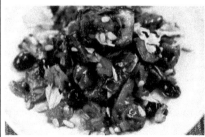

✓ The nutritional facts: calories 170, fat 13, fiber 3, carbs 5, protein 7

RUTABAGA AND CHERRY TOMATOES MIX

Prep. time: 10 minutes The cooking time: 15 minutes The recipe servings: 4

Fixings	Guidelines
❖ 1 tablespoon shallot, hacked ❖ 1 garlic clove, minced ❖ ¾ cup cashews, splashed for a few hours and depleted ❖ 2 tablespoons The nutritional factsal yeast ❖ ½ cup veggie stock ❖ Salt and dark pepper to the taste ❖ 2 teaspoons lemon juice ❖ For the pasta:	➤ Place tomatoes and rutabaga noodles into a container that accommodates the air fryer cooker, shower the oil over them, season with salt, dark pepper and garlic powder, hurl to cover and cook in the air fryer cooker at 350 Deg. Fahrenheit for about 15 minutes. ➤ Meanwhile, in a food processor, blend garlic in with shallots, cashews, veggie stock, The nutritional factsal yeast, lemon squeeze, a spot of ocean salt and dark pepper to the taste and mix well. ➤ Divide rutabaga pasta on plates, top with tomatoes,

	sprinkle the sauce over them and serve.
❖ cup cherry tomatoes, divided	Enjoy the recipe!
❖ 5 teaspoons olive oil	
❖ ¼ teaspoon garlic powder	
❖ rutabagas, stripped and cut into thick noodles	

✓ The nutritional facts: calories 160, fat 2, fiber 5, carbs 10, protein 8

GARLIC TOMATOES

Prep. time: 10 minutes: The cooking time: 15 minutes: The recipe servings: 4

Fixings	Guidelines
❖ 4 garlic cloves, squashed	➢ In a bowl, blend tomatoes in with salt, dark pepper, garlic, olive oil and thyme, hurl to cover, present in the air fryer cooker and cook at 360 Deg. Fahrenheit for about 15 minutes.
❖ 1 pound blended cherry tomatoes	
❖ 3 thyme springs, hacked	
❖ Salt and dark pepper to the taste	➢ Divide tomatoes blend on plates and serve.

❖ ¼ cup olive oil	Enjoy the recipe!

✓ The nutritional facts: calories 100, fat 0, fiber 1, carbs 1, protein 6

TOMATO AND BASIL TART

Prep. time: 10 minutes: The cooking time: 14 minutes: The recipe servings: 2

Fixings	Guidelines
❖ 1 bundle basil, hacked ❖ 4 eggs ❖ garlic clove, minced ❖ Salt and dark pepper to the taste ❖ ½ cup cherry tomatoes, divided ❖ ¼ cup cheddar, ground	➤ In a bowl, blend eggs in with salt, dark pepper, cheddar and basil and whisk well. ➤ Pour this into a heating dish that accommodates the air fryer cooker, mastermind tomatoes on top, present in the fryer and cook at 320 Deg. Fahrenheit for about 14 minutes. ➤ Slice and serve immediately. Enjoy the recipe!

✓ The nutritional facts: calories 140, fat 1, fiber 1, carbs 2, protein 10

ZUCCHINI NOODLES DELIGHT

Prep. time: 10 minutes: The cooking time: 20 minutes: The recipe servings: 6

Fixings	Guidelines
❖ 2tablespoons olive oil ❖ 2 zucchinis, cut with a spiralizer ❖ 16 ounces mushrooms, cut ❖ ¼ cup sun dried tomatoes, cleaved ❖ 1 teaspoon garlic, minced ❖ ½ cup cherry tomatoes, divided ❖ 2 cups tomatoes sauce ❖ 2 cups spinach, torn ❖ Salt and dark pepper to the taste ❖ A bunch basil, cleaved	➢ Put zucchini noodles in a bowl, season salt and dark pepper and leave them aside for 10 minutes. ➢ Heat up a container that accommodates the air fryer cooker with the oil over medium high heat, include garlic, mix and cook for 1 moment. ➢ Add mushrooms, sun dried tomatoes, cherry tomatoes, spinach, cayenne, sauce and zucchini noodles, mix, present in the air fryer cooker and cook at 320 Deg. Fahrenheit for about 10 minutes. ➢ Divide among plates and present with basil sprinkled on top .Enjoy the recipe!

✓ The nutritional facts: calories 120, fat 1, fiber 1, carbs 2, protein 9

BASIC TOMATOES AND BELL PEPPER SAUCE

Prep. time: 10 minutes: The cooking time: 15 minutes: The recipe servings: 4

Fixings	Guidelines
❖ 2 red ringer peppers, slashed ❖ 2 garlic cloves, minced ❖ 1 pound cherry tomatoes, divided ❖ 1 teaspoon rosemary, dried ❖ 3 straight leaves ❖ 2 tablespoons olive oil ❖ 1 tablespoon balsamic vinegar ❖ Salt and dark pepper to the taste	➢ In a bowl blend tomatoes in with garlic, salt, dark pepper, rosemary, straight leaves, half of the oil and half of the vinegar, hurl to cover, present in the air fryer cooker and meal them at 320 Deg. Fahrenheit for about 15 minutes. ➢ Meanwhile, in your food processor, blend ringer peppers with a spot of ocean salt, dark pepper, the remainder of the oil and the remainder of the vinegar and mix well indeed. ➢ Divide cooked tomatoes on plates, shower the chime peppers sauce over them and serve. Enjoy the recipe!

✓ The nutritional facts: calories 123, fat 1, fiber 1, carbs 8, protein 10

CHERRY TOMATOES SKEWERS

Prep. time: 10 minutes: The cooking time: 6 minutes: The recipe servings: 4

Fixings	Guidelines
❖ 3 tablespoons balsamic vinegar 24 cherry tomatoes ❖ Tablespoons thyme, cleaved ❖ Salt and dark pepper to the taste ❖ For the dressing: ❖ tablespoons balsamic vinegar ❖ Salt and dark pepper to the taste ❖ 4 tablespoons olive oil	➢ In a bowl, blend 2 tablespoons oil with 3 tablespoons vinegar, 3 garlic cloves, thyme, salt and dark pepper and whisk well. ➢ Add tomatoes, hurl to cover and leave aside for 30 minutes. ➢ Arrange 6 tomatoes on one stick and rehash with the remainder of the tomatoes. ➢ Introduce them in the air fryer cooker and cook at 360 Deg. Fahrenheit for about 6 minutes.

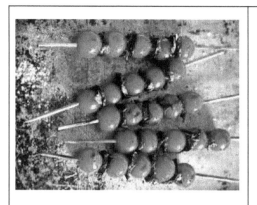

> In another bowl, blend 2 tablespoons vinegar in with salt, pepper and 4 tablespoons oil and whisk well.

> Arrange tomato sticks on plates and present with the dressing showered on top.

Enjoy the recipe!

✓ The nutritional facts: calories 140, fat 1, fiber 1, carbs 2, protein 7

FLAVORFUL PORTOBELLO MUSHROOMS

Prep. time: 10 minutes: The cooking time: 12 minutes: The recipe servings: 4

Fixings	Guidelines
❖ 10 basil leaves ❖ 1 cup infant spinach ❖ 3 garlic cloves, slashed	> In your food processor, blend basil in with spinach, garlic, almonds, parsley, oil, salt, dark pepper to the taste and mushroom stems and mix well.

❖ 1 cup almonds, generally slashed	➢ Stuff each mushroom with this blend, place them in the air fryer cooker and cook at 350 Deg. Fahrenheit for about 12 minutes.
❖ 1 tablespoon parsley	
❖ ¼ cup olive oil	➢ Divide mushrooms on plates and serve.
❖ 8 cherry tomatoes, divided	
❖ Salt and dark pepper to the taste	Enjoy the recipe!
❖ 4 Portobello mushrooms, stems evacuated and slashed	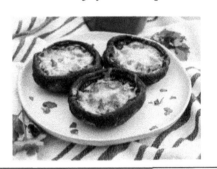

✓ The nutritional facts: calories 145, fat 3, fiber 2, carbs 6, protein 17

MEXICAN PEPPERS

Prep. time: 10 minutes: The cooking time: 25 minutes: The recipe servings: 4

Fixings	Guidelines
❖ ringer peppers, finishes cut off and seeds evacuated ❖ ½ cup tomato juice	➢ In a skillet that accommodates the air fryer cooker, blend chicken bosoms in with tomato juice, jalapenos, tomatoes, onion, green peppers, salt, pepper, onion powder, red pepper,

- ❖ 2 tablespoons jostled jalapenos, hacked

- ❖ 4 chicken bosoms

- ❖ 1 cup tomatoes, hacked

- ❖ ¼ cup yellow onion, slashed

- ❖ ¼ cup green peppers, slashed

- ❖ 2 cups tomato sauce

- ❖ Salt and dark pepper to the taste

- ❖ 2 teaspoons onion powder

- ❖ ½ teaspoon red pepper, squashed

- ❖ 1 teaspoon bean stew powder

- ❖ ½ teaspoons garlic powder

- ❖ 1 teaspoon cumin, ground

stew powder, garlic powder, oregano and cumin, mix well, present in the air fryer cooker and cook at 350 Deg. Fahrenheit for about 15 minutes,

➢ Shred meat utilizing 2 forks, mix, stuff ringer peppers with this blend, place them in the air fryer cooker and cook at 320 Deg. Fahrenheit for about 10 minutes more.

➢ Divide stuffed peppers on plates and serve.

Enjoy the recipe!

✓ The nutritional facts: calories 180, fat 4, fiber 3, carbs 7, protein 14

PEPPERS STUFFED WITH BEEF

Prep. time: 10 minutes: The cooking time: 55 minutes: The recipe servings: 4

Fixings	Guidelines
❖ 1 pound hamburger, ground ❖ 1 teaspoon coriander, ground 1 onion, slashed ❖ 3 garlic cloves, minced & 2 tablespoonful of olive oil ❖ 1 tablespoon ginger, ground ❖ ½ teaspoon cumin, ground ❖ ½ teaspoon turmeric powder ❖ 1 tablespoon hot curry powder ❖ Salt and dark pepper to	➢ Heat up a skillet with the oil over medium high heat, include onion, mix and cook for 4 minutes. ➢ Add garlic and hamburger, mix and cook for 10 minutes. ➢ Add coriander, ginger, cumin, curry powder, salt, pepper, turmeric, pecans and raisins, mix take off heat and blend in with the egg. ➢ Stuff pepper parts with this blend, present them in the air fryer cooker and cook at 320 Deg. Fahrenheit for about 20 minutes. ➢ Divide among plates and serve.

the taste	Enjoy the recipe
❖ 1 egg	
❖ 4 ringer peppers, cut into equal parts and seeds evacuated	
❖ 1/3 cup raisins	
❖ 1/3 cup pecans, slashed	

✓ The nutritional facts: calories 170, fat 4, fiber 3, carbs 7, protein 12

STUFFED POBLANO PEPPERS

Prep. time: 10 minutes: The cooking time: 15 minutes: The recipe servings: 4

Fixings	Guidelines
❖ 2teaspoons garlic, minced ❖ 1 white onion, slashed ❖ 10 poblano peppers, finishes cut off and deseeded ❖ 1 tablespoon of olive oil ❖ 8 ounces mushrooms,	➢ Heat up a skillet with the oil over medium high heat, include onion and mushrooms, mix and cook for 5 minutes. ➢ Add garlic, cilantro, salt and dark pepper, mix and cook for 2 minutes. ➢ Divide this blend into

slashed ❖ Salt and dark pepper to the taste ❖ ½ cup cilantro, slashed 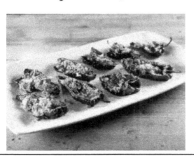	poblanos, present them in the air fryer cooker and cook at 350 Deg. Fahrenheit for about 15 minutes. ➢ Divide among plates and serve. Enjoy the recipe!

✓ The nutritional facts: calories 150, fat 3, fiber 2, carbs 7, protein 10

STUFFED BABY PEPPERS

Prep. time: 10 minutes: The cooking time: 6 minutes: The recipe servings: 4

Fixings	Guidelines
❖ 12 infant ringer peppers, cut into equal parts the long way ❖ ¼ teaspoon red pepper pieces, squashed ❖ 1 pound shrimp, cooked, stripped and deveined	➢ In a bowl, blend shrimp in with pepper pieces, pesto, salt, dark pepper, lemon juice, oil and parsley, whisk well indeed and stuff chime pepper parts with this blend. ➢ Place them in the air fryer cooker and cook at 320

❖ 6 tablespoons jolted basil pesto	Deg. Fahrenheit for about 6 minutes,
❖ Salt and dark pepper to the taste	➢ Arrange peppers on plates and serve.
❖ 1 tablespoon lemon juice	
❖ tablespoon of olive oil	Enjoy the recipe!
❖ A bunch parsley, hacked	

✓ The nutritional facts: calories 130, fat 2, fiber 1, carbs 3, protein 15

EGGPLANT AND GARLIC SAUCE

Prep. time: 10 minutes: The cooking time: 10 minutes: The recipe servings: 4

Fixings	Guidelines
❖ 2tablespoons olive oil ❖ 2 garlic cloves, minced ❖ 2 eggplants, split and cut 1 red stew pepper, slashed ❖ 1 green onion stalk, hacked ❖ 1tablespoon ginger, ground	➢ Heat up a dish that accommodates the air fryer cooker with the oil over medium high heat, include eggplant cuts and cook for 2 minutes. ➢ Add stew pepper, garlic, green onions, ginger, soy sauce and vinegar, present in the air fryer cooker and cook at 320 Deg.

❖ 1 tablespoon soy sauce ❖ 1 tablespoon balsamic vinegar	Fahrenheit for about 7 minutes. ➢ Divide among plates and serve. Enjoy the recipe!

✓ The nutritional facts: calories 130, fat 2, fiber 4, carbs 7, protein 9

EGGPLANT HASH

Prep. time: 20 minutes: The cooking time: 10 minutes: The recipe servings: 4

Fixings	Guidelines
❖ 1 eggplant, generally cleaved ❖ ½ cup olive oil ❖ ½ pound cherry tomatoes, divided ❖ 1 teaspoon Tabasco sauce ❖ ¼ cup basil, cleaved ❖ ¼ cup mint, cleaved	➢ Heat up a container that accommodates the air fryer cooker with half of the oil over medium high heat, include eggplant pieces, cook for 3 minutes, flip, cook them for 3 minutes more and move to a bowl. ➢ Heat up a similar dish with the remainder of the oil over medium high heat, include tomatoes, mix and cook for 1-2 minutes.

❖ Salt and dark pepper to the taste 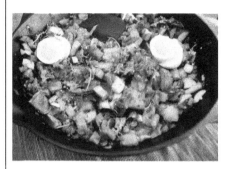	➢ Return eggplant pieces to the skillet, include salt, dark pepper, basil, mint and Tabasco sauce, present in the air fryer cooker and cook at 320 Deg. Fahrenheit for about 6 minutes. ➢ Divide among plates and serve. Enjoy the recipe!

✓ The nutritional facts: calories 120, fat 1, fiber 4, carbs 8, protein 15

SWEET POTATOES MIX

Prep. time: 10 minutes: The cooking time: 15 minutes: The recipe servings: 4

Fixings	Guidelines
❖ 3 sweet potatoes, cubed, 4 garlic cloves, minced ❖ ½ pound bacon, slashed Juice from 1 lime ❖ Salt and dark pepper to the taste 2 tablespoons	➢ Arrange bacon and sweet potatoes in the air fryer cooker's container, include garlic and half of the oil, hurl well and cook at 350 degrees F and prepare for 15 minutes. ➢ Meanwhile, in a bowl, blend vinegar in with lime juice,

balsamic vinegar A bunch dill, slashed

❖ 2 green onions, slashed

❖ A spot of cinnamon powder A touch of red pepper pieces | olive oil, green onions, pepper drops, dill, salt, pepper and cinnamon and whisk.

➢ Transfer bacon and sweet potatoes to a plate of mixed greens bowl, include plate of mixed greens dressing, hurl well and serve immediately.

Enjoy the recipe! |

✓ The nutritional facts: calories 170, fat 3, fiber 2, carbs 5, protein 12

GREEK POTATO MIX

Prep. time: 10 minutes: The cooking time: 20 minutes: The recipe servings: 2

Fixings	Guidelines
❖ 2 medium potatoes, cut into wedges

❖ 1 yellow onion, hacked

❖ 2 tablespoons spread

❖ 1 little carrot, generally hacked | ➢ Heat up a dish that accommodates the air fryer cooker with the spread over medium high heat, include onion and carrot, mix and cook for 3-4 minutes.

➢ Add potatoes, flour, chicken stock, salt, pepper and sound leaf, mix, |

❖ 1 and ½ tablespoon flour	present in the air fryer cooker and cook at 320 Deg. Fahrenheit for about 16 minutes.
❖ bay leaf	
❖ ½ cup chicken stock	➢ Add Greek yogurt, hurl, separate among plates and serve.
❖ tablespoons Greek yogurt	
❖ Salt and dark pepper to the taste	Enjoy the recipe!

✓ The nutritional facts: calories 198, fat 3, fiber 2, carbs 6, protein

BROCCOLI HASH

Prep. time: 30 minutes: The cooking time: 8 minutes: The recipe servings: 2

Fixings	Guidelines
❖ 10 ounces mushrooms, divided	➢ In a bowl, blend mushrooms in with broccoli, onion, garlic and avocado.
❖ 1 broccoli head, florets isolated	
❖ 1 garlic clove, minced	➢ In another bowl, blend vinegar, oil, salt, pepper and basil and whisk well.
❖ 1 tablespoon balsamic vinegar	➢ Pour this over veggies, hurl

❖ 1 yellow onion, hacked	to cover, leave aside for 30 minutes, move to the air fryer cooker's bin and cook at 350 Deg. Fahrenheit for about 8 minutes,
❖ 1 tablespoon of olive oil Salt and dark pepper	
❖ 1 teaspoon basil, dried	➢ Divide among plates and present with pepper pieces on top.
❖ avocado, stripped and pitted	
❖ A spot of red pepper chips	Enjoy the recipe!

✓ The nutritional facts: calories 182, fat 3, fiber 3, carbs 5, protein 8

AIR FRIED ASPARAGUS

Prep. time: 10 minutes: The cooking time: 15 minutes: The recipe servings: 4

Fixings	Rules
❖ 2pounds crisp asparagus, cut	➢ In a bowl, blend oil in with lemon pizzazz, garlic, pepper chips and oregano and whisk.
❖ ¼ cup olive oil	
❖ Salt and dark pepper to the taste	➢ Add asparagus, cheddar, salt and pepper, hurl, move to the air fryer cooker's container and cook at 350

❖ 1 teaspoon lemon pizzazz	Deg. Fahrenheit for about 8 minutes.
❖ 4 garlic cloves, minced	
❖ ½ teaspoon oregano, dried	➢ Partition asparagus on plates, shower lemon squeeze and sprinkle parsley on top and serve.
❖ ¼ teaspoon red pepper pieces	
	Enjoy the recipe!
❖ 4 ounces feta cheddar, disintegrated	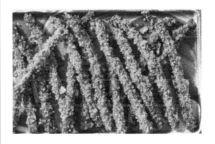
❖ 2 tablespoons parsley, finely cleaved Juice from 1 lemon	

✓ The nutritional facts: calories 162, fat 13, fiber 5, carbs 12, protein 8

STUFFED EGGPLANTS

Prep. time: 10 minutes: The cooking time: 30 minutes: The recipe servings: 4

Fixings	Rules
❖ 4 little eggplants, split the long way ❖ Salt and dark pepper to the taste	➢ Season eggplants with salt, pepper and 4 tablespoons oil, hurl, put them in the air fryer cooker and cook at 350 Deg. Fahrenheit for about 16 minutes.

- ❖ 10 tablespoons olive oil

- ❖ 2 and ½ pounds tomatoes, cut into equal parts and ground

- ❖ 1 green ringer pepper, hacked

- ❖ 1 yellow onion, cleaved

- ❖ 1 tablespoon garlic, minced

- ❖ ½ cup cauliflower, cleaved

- ❖ 1 teaspoon oregano, slashed

- ❖ ½ cup parsley, cleaved

- ❖ 3 ounces feta cheddar, disintegrated

- ➢ Meanwhile, heat up a container with 3 tablespoons oil over medium high heat, include onion, mix and cook for 5 minutes.

- ➢ Add chime pepper, garlic and cauliflower, mix, cook for 5 minutes, take off heat, include parsley, tomato, salt, pepper, oregano and cheddar and whisk everything.

- ➢ Stuff eggplants with the veggie blend, shower the remainder of the oil over them, put them in the air fryer cooker and cook at 350 Deg. Fahrenheit for about 6 minutes more.

- ➢ Divide among plates and serve immediately.

Enjoy the formula!

- ✓ The nutritional facts: calories 240, fat 4, fiber, 2, carbs 19, protein 2

GREEN BEANS AND PARMESAN

Prep. time: 10 minutes: The cooking time: 8 minutes: The recipe servings: 4

Fixings	Rules
❖ 12 ounces green beans	➢ In a bowl, blend oil in with salt, pepper, garlic and egg and whisk well.
❖ 2 teaspoons of garlic, minced with	
❖ 2 tablespoons olive oil	➢ Add green beans to this blend, hurl well and sprinkle parmesan everywhere.
❖ Salt and dark pepper to the taste	➢ Transfer green beans to the air fryer cooker and cook them at 390 Deg. Fahrenheit for about 8 minutes.
❖ 1 egg, whisked	
❖ 1/3 cup parmesan, ground	➢ Divide green beans on plates and serve them immediately.
	Enjoy the formula!

✓ The nutritional facts: calories 120, fat 8, fiber 2, carbs 7, protein 4

TASTY CREAMY GREEN BEANS

Prep. time: 10 minutes: The cooking time: 15 minutes: The recipe servings: 4

Fixings	Rules
❖ ½ cup overwhelming cream ❖ cup mozzarella, destroyed ❖ 2/3 cup parmesan, ground ❖ Salt and dark pepper to the taste ❖ 2 pounds green beans ❖ teaspoons lemon get-up-and-go, ground ❖ A spot of red pepper pieces	➢ Put the beans in a dish that accommodates the air fryer cooker, include overwhelming cream, salt, pepper, lemon pizzazz, pepper pieces, mozzarella and parmesan, hurl, present in the air fryer cooker and cook at 350 Deg. Fahrenheit for about 15 minutes. ➢ Divide among plates and serve immediately. Enjoy the formula!

✓ The nutritional facts: calories 231, fat 6, fiber 7, carbs 8, protein 5

GREEN BEANS AND TOMATOES

Prep. time: 10 minutes: The cooking time: 15 minutes: The recipe servings: 4

Fixings	Rules
❖ 1pint cherry tomatoes ❖ 1 pound green beans ❖ ❖ tablespoons olive oil ❖ Salt and dark pepper to the taste	➤ In a bowl, blend cherry tomatoes in with green beans, olive oil, salt and pepper, hurl, move to the air fryer cooker and cook at 400 Deg. Fahrenheit for about 15 minutes. ➤ Divide among plates and serve immediately. Enjoy the formula!

✓ The nutritional facts: calories 162, fat 6, fiber 5, carbs 8, protein 9

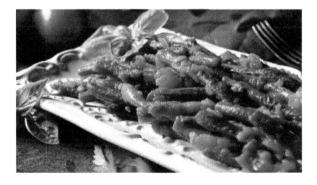

SIMPLE GREEN BEANS AND POTATOES

Prep. time: 10 minutes: The cooking time: 15 minutes: The recipe
servings: 5

Fixings	Rules
❖ 2 pounds green beans ❖ 6 new potatoes, split ❖ Salt and dark pepper to the taste A shower of olive oil ❖ 6 bacon cuts, cooked and hacked	➢ In a bowl, blend green beans in with potatoes, salt, pepper and oil, hurl, move to the air fryer cooker and cook at 390 Deg. Fahrenheit for about 15 minutes. ➢ Divide among plates and present with bacon sprinkled on top. Enjoy the formula!

✓ The nutritional facts: calories 374, fat 15, fiber 12, carbs 28, protein 12

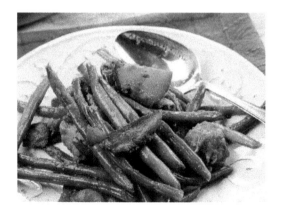

ENHANCED GREEN BEANS

Prep. time: 10 minutes: The cooking time: 15minutes: The recipe servings: 4

Fixings	Rules
❖ 1pound red potatoes, cut into wedges ❖ 1 pound green beans ❖ garlic cloves, minced ❖ 2 tablespoons olive oil ❖ Salt and dark pepper to the taste ❖ ½ teaspoon oregano, dried	➢ In a skillet that accommodates the air fryer cooker, consolidate potatoes with green beans, garlic, oil, salt, pepper and oregano, hurl, present in the air fryer cooker and cook at 380 Deg. Fahrenheit for about 15 minutes. ➢ Divide among plates and serve. Enjoy the formula!

✓ The nutritional facts: calories 211, fat 6, fiber 7, carbs 8, protein 5

POTATOES AND TOMATOES MIX

Prep. time: 10 minutes: The cooking time: 16 minutes: The recipe servings: 4

Fixings	Rules
❖ 1 and ½ pounds red potatoes, quartered ❖ 2 tablespoons olive oil ❖ 1 16 ounces cherry tomatoes ❖ 1 teaspoon sweet paprika ❖ 1 tablespoons rosemary, cleaved ❖ Salt and dark pepper to the taste ❖ 3 garlic cloves, minced	➤ In a bowl, blend potatoes in with tomatoes, oil, paprika, rosemary, garlic, salt and pepper, hurl, move to the air fryer cooker and cook at 380 Deg. Fahrenheit for about 16 minutes. ➤ Divide among plates and serve. Enjoy the formula!

✓ The nutritional facts: calories 192, fat 4, fiber 4, carbs 30, protein 3

BALSAMIC POTATOES

Prep. time: 10 minutes The cooking time: 20 minutes The recipe servings: 4

Fixings	Rules
❖ and ½ pounds infant potatoes, split	➤ In your food processor, blend garlic in with onions, oil, vinegar, thyme, salt and pepper and heartbeat truly well.
❖ 2 garlic cloves, slashed	
❖ red onions, cleaved	
❖ 9 ounces cherry tomatoes	➤ In a bowl, blend potatoes in with tomatoes and balsamic marinade, hurl well, move to the air fryer cooker and cook at 380 Deg. Fahrenheit for about 20 minutes.
❖ 3 tablespoons olive oil	
❖ and ½ tablespoons balsamic vinegar	➤ Divide among plates and serve.
❖ 2 thyme springs, cleaved	
❖ Salt and dark pepper to the taste	Enjoy the formula!

✓ The nutritional facts: calories 301, fat 6, fiber 8, carbs 18, protein 6

POTATOES AND SPECIAL TOMATO SAUCE

Prep. time: 10 minutes The cooking time: 16 minutes The recipe servings: 4

Fixings	Rules
❖ 2 pounds potatoes, cubed ❖ 4 garlic cloves, minced ❖ yellow onion, hacked ❖ 1 cup tomato sauce ❖ tablespoons basil, hacked ❖ 2 tablespoons olive oil ❖ ½ teaspoon oregano, dried ❖ ½ teaspoon parsley, dried	➢ Heat up a dish that accommodates the air fryer cooker with the oil over medium heat, include onion, mix and cook for 1-2 minutes. ➢ Add garlic, potatoes, parsley, tomato sauce and oregano, mix, present in the air fryer cooker and cook at 370 degrees F and cook for 16 minutes. ➢ Add basil, hurl everything, separate among plates and serve. Enjoy the formula!

✓ The nutritional facts: calories 211, fat 6, fiber 8, carbs 14, protein 6

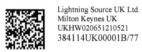